HIV, AIDS and Children
A Cause for Concern

by

by Naomi Honigsbaum

Funded by a grant from the National AIDS Trust and Action for
Children, National Children's Bureau and The Wellcome Foundation Ltd

ISBN 0 902 817 63 9

Published by the National Children's Bureau
8 Wakley Street
London EC1V 7QE
Telephone 071 278 9441

Reprinted October 1991.

Typeset, printed and bound by Saxon Printing Ltd, Derby.

The National Children's Bureau was established as a registered charity in
1963. Our purpose is to identify and promote the interests of all children
and young people and to improve their status in a diverse and multiracial
society.

We work closely with professionals and policy makers to improve the lives
of all children but especially children under five, those affected by family
instability and children with special needs or disabilities.

We collect and disseminate information about children and promote good
practice in children's services through research, policy and practice
development, publications, seminars, training and an extensive library
and information service

HIV, AIDS and Children
A Cause for Concern

Contents

Part III

Acknowledgements

I would like to thank all those who gave generously of their time, expertise and knowledge in helping me to compile the material for this report, including those who completed the questionnaire.

In particular, I would like to thank the resident women and children of Brenda House for their hospitality and courage, Terry Cotton of the HIV Unit, London Borough of Hammersmith and Fulham and Philippa Russell of the Voluntary Council for Handicapped Children for her valuable guidance and support throughout the project, and Jane Holden of Elliott-Holden Editing for her editorial comments.

Naomi Honigsbaum
February 1991

Foreword

The World Health Organisation has recently predicted that by the
end of the decade 10 million children will have AIDS and another 10
million will have been orphaned by the HIV virus. These global
figures, which, sadly, are probably an underestimate, reflect the
scale of the worldwide problem which all of us concerned with AIDS
and the family will have to confront.

In the UK we are, at the moment, dealing with numbers in the
hundreds rather than the millions and, although the epidemic will
undoubtedly grow, we still have time to plan our responses and
organise our services in a way which may prevent an explosive
increase in infection and provide the most efficient, compassionate
care for all those affected.

In both the developing and the industrial world, the link between
family poverty and HIV/AIDS is increasingly becoming more firmly
established. In the villages of Africa, the inner cities of the United
States and, increasingly, in Europe, the spread of AIDS is now
identified as a phenomenon of multiple deprivation. This has had
particular significance for family policy in societies like ours where
more and more mothers are single parents and family wage earners.
These women and children already feel isolated and stigmatised and
the discrimination associated with HIV compounds a sense of
alienation which makes it very difficult for them to accept information or help from outside. AIDS is the 'last straw' in lives afflicted by
every kind of social and material disadvantage.

In Britain, our National Health Service and social service
networks, combined with well-established family and voluntary
childcare organisations, should provide a framework for combating
the new threat of AIDS. This report, *HIV, AIDS and Children – A*

Cause for Concern, demonstrates, disturbingly, that most of those best placed to develop services have yet to give high priority to this issue.

Many people working with children, often with scarce resources and with many competing professional pressures, still see HIV and AIDS as a marginal problem. This report is very timely in identifying immediate needs, offering an agenda for policy and practice to meet future needs, and addressing the complex emotional and ethical issues which often inhibit action in this very sensitive area.

All of this will, as the report acknowledges, require extra resources, special training and above all collaboration between agencies from different professional backgrounds. It would be naively unrealistic to expect rapid and radical change, but what is hopeful about HIV/AIDS and children is that the basic structures for implementing new strategies already exist. So often in the brief history of AIDS, unfamiliar issues confronting different groups of people have required fresh responses from different organisations, but childcare is provided for by a multitude of well-established mechanisms. There is no need to invent or re-invent the wheel, simply to modify and extend it to encompass the special issues of HIV/AIDS. From the perspective of the National AIDS Trust, which is primarily a voluntary sector development agency, it has been particularly encouraging to see how energetically agencies such as the National Children's Bureau, Barnardo's and Save the Children Fund are using their skills to tackle HIV/AIDS. There is a wealth of talent and a long record of pioneering work with families and children to be drawn on when we all face up to the wide impact of the epidemic.

Naomi Honigsbaum's report underlines the crucial importance of a child-centred approach in creating AIDS strategies. The philosophy has underpinned most children's policy in this country for many years, but it must be vigilantly guarded and monitored in an area where human rights, confidentiality and personal wishes have been so badly threatened. The key principle of the Children Act is to 'listen to children' and this must be not just our pious hope, but our practical touchstone in all the thinking and planning which needs urgently to be started.

In the nineties we need to be able to care adequately for all those children who are affected by HIV/AIDS and to ensure that the 21st century does not begin with an unnecessary legacy of preventable infection. I welcome this report as an essential step towards achieving those goals.

Margaret Jay
Director, National AIDS Trust
March 1991

Part I

Preface

'Some children are being treated like social pariahs. I recently heard of a boy of 14 years who was confined to his room because he had HIV.'
Welfare benefits worker

'They told me quite casually that I was HIV, there was no warning, and there I was just left alone to deal with the emotional shock and horror. What I wanted was someone to sit down and treat me like a human being.'
Young woman

'After the baby was born I was left alone in a room by myself, the baby wasn't weighed for several hours because they hadn't disinfected the scales.'
Mother

'The parents just refuse to tell him that he is infected, and insist that he mustn't know. I think he knows – children are very quick to sense these things; the 'hushed tones'; all these tests and treatments – it's the parents who don't want to know.'
Nurse in Haemophilia Centre

'I know my children are worried, sometimes they ask me if I'm going to die, or if they are going to die. I just won't talk about it, I try not to mention it at all. I really don't know what they understand.'
Mother

'I just wouldn't go to social services when I knew I was pregnant, because I thought they'd try to take the baby away from me.'
Former drug user

'Anyway, if I did contract HIV at work, would I get any compensation?'
Residential care worker

'I would like to know how to talk to this mother about her child who has HIV. She's very intelligent, but she refuses to discuss it – it's very difficult to counsel her.'
Headteacher

'Some school dentists don't seem to understand the difference between HIV infection and haemophilia'.
Doctor, DHA

'I learnt I was HIV because of the special marks on my case notes, which I read.'
Mother

'When they're on the streets – homeless and with no money – its no good talking to them about safer sex and asserting yourself, or handing out condoms and free needles; their main priority is finding somewhere to sleep for the night, not protecting themselves.'
Worker with outreach project

'She doesn't speak English and I have to communicate with her by drawing diagrams, she has no family here and is very ill.'
Social worker

1. Introduction

What exactly do we know about the range and quality of services currently provided for children with HIV infection and AIDS, and are we making adequate provision for future needs if the rate of infection increases and the patterns and prevalence change? Are there unmet needs now, and if so, what are the implications for the future development and planning of childcare policies and services?

In order to answer some of these questions the National Children's Bureau was financed by the National AIDS Trust to undertake a mapping exercise to identify the major issues and current initiatives in relation to HIV services for children. This book is the result of that inquiry.

The comments and thoughts of individuals which open this book illustrate graphically the daily indignities and profoundly distressing experiences that still appear commonplace for children with HIV infection and their families and carers. They also highlight the range of professional and organisational dilemmas, and the confusion which is aroused in any attempt to identify:

- clear policy and practice goals;
- coordinated and coherent approaches to service planning for children;
- child and family-centred policies which are qualitatively life-enhancing and sensitive.

This book attempts to address some of these concerns and suggests ways in which services need to adjust and change in order to reflect a more child-centred approach. Information and material was compiled from a postal survey questionnaire, seminars, interviews, visits and a literature search.

The aim of the study was to identify the current issues, concerns and initiatives in HIV related services for children by looking at professional, statutory and voluntary sector provision in health, education and the personal social services. Children were defined (for the purposes of the study) as those within the 0–18-year-old range, but because policies and services are also directed at 16–25-year-olds, some overlap was inevitable. Whilst the primary focus was on children, it was not possible to consider their needs in isolation from those of their families, carers and extended networks. This was particularly relevant as the study raised many concerns and worries about the low socio-economic conditions of families with HIV infected children and highlights the need to review social policies and provision for these families.

Overview

This overview introduces briefly the major themes that emerged from this study. These themes are then explored in greater depth and the book offers, in summation, recommendations for future development and improvements.

It is impossible to forecast the future spread of HIV infection and AIDS in the child population in the UK with any degree of certainty. Consequently the planning of services for children will have to continue to rely for some time on 'soft' information.[1] These uncertainties may frustrate and discourage statutory and voluntary bodies from taking a more proactive stance in developing HIV related services for children. Yet any delays in *beginning* this process will be detrimental, in the long run, to the quality and range of services provided for children and their families. The study identified a common view that HIV services should not be considered in isolation from the overall goals of an organisation – they should be addressed within the context of the development of good childcare practice.

Considerable unease and criticism was directed at central government throughout the study. It was felt that the government was abrogating its role in developing a set of clear principles and guidance in relation to HIV childcare issues. There is serious cause for concern about the poor quality of much childcare practice – children are often vulnerable and in a powerless role in relation to the adults who care for them. It was felt that government should be more proactive in setting standards, developing monitoring systems and targeting resources for the front-line agencies. It was feared that the thrust of current policy changes and legislation in health, education and social services could lead to greater fragmentation of children's services. This highlighted the importance of maintaining an overview on planning mechanisms and questioning whether appropriate structures existed across organisational boundaries for developing coordinated childcare strategies.

There is a need to question fundamentally many current professional attitudes and approaches to childcare practice. Ideally childcare strategies and practice should be underpinned by a philosophy that recognises the *inherent* rights and autonomy of children and seeks actively to involve them and their families in all aspects and decisions about their welfare. Many services for children need to review their approach and develop a more child-centred focus – to encourage attitudes which are not patronising. In organisations where the primary focus is on direct work with children, staff should be especially trained in the skills and techniques of communicating with all children, including those with special needs. Agencies should be more imaginative in developing a variety of written and illustrated information and educational material that is age-related and reflects the ethnic origins and cultural differences of children.

It has to be acknowledged that some childcare practices are quite appalling. The study revealed some accounts of distressing and humiliating treatment of young people by adults that need to be investigated. Many staff still appear to lack even basic knowledge and understanding about HIV transmission. This ignorance can sometimes lead to bizarre, cruel and stigmatising behaviour by staff towards a young person who may be HIV positive. Developing appropriate policies and training on HIV still seems to lag far behind the rhetoric.

There are great regional variations in the pattern and distribution of services for children with HIV infection. In many ways it mirrors similar experiences of how services evolved for adults with HIV in response to local needs. At present most experience has been developed in centres such as Edinburgh which has the largest identified group of HIV infected children, and in some London districts and haemophilia centres. With the exception of these centres, most organisations and professional staff may as yet have had only minimal experience of or involvement with infected children. The survey revealed that professional staff often felt socially isolated and unsure in their own knowledge base and skills in relation to the care and treatment of children with HIV. Many staff commented that they had been given no clear guidance or training and often felt the lack of staff support or a forum within the organisation in which to raise these issues. There was often little understanding of the roles of other disciplines both within agencies and across agency boundaries, and some confusion and rivalry about which staff group has key responsibility. For example, who in the school setting is responsible for health education? Is it the teacher, school nurse or drugs coordinator? Most of the services for children with HIV were, primarily, being developed around a health care model – such as haemophilia centres and paediatric hospital departments. Some social service departments have pioneered models of shared care and have developed comprehensive training programmes and policy guidance for foster/adoptive parents and childcare staff. These models support parents in caring for a sick child but also provide respite care or foster care when parents need additional help or relief, or when they themselves become ill.

Initiatives have been developed by voluntary childcare bodies such as National Foster Care Association, Preschool Playgroup Association and Save the Children Fund which have promoted HIV awareness and training for staff, and emphasised the importance of educating parents and carers. These educational initiatives aim to ensure that children with HIV infection are not rejected because of fears of transmission and are integrated into normal childcare programmes.

There is concern that many of the smaller voluntary organisations who work in community out-reach projects, street agencies, drug services and drop-in centres are grossly under-resourced. They are also less likely to *attract* adequate funding, even though they are more likely to be in touch with needy young people and families who are at risk of contracting HIV or may already be infected. These services should be adequately funded as they work with the more difficult and hard to reach young people – a group who will not seek help from the more traditional services. Staff working with vulnerable young people were only too well aware of the frustrating and inherent contradictions in much of their work. Encouraging young people to take better care of their health seems pointless to staff if they have no alternative to sleeping 'rough' on the streets – or to prostitution in return for a night's food and shelter.

The needs of children with HIV cannot easily be considered separately from the needs of their families and their cultural, religious and ethnic backgrounds. There is a particular relationship between the needs of children and the role of women as parents and carers. Many of the recommendations in this study emphasise the need to support the *family* in its caring role by providing improved and accessible services which are responsive to local situations. This need will have major implications for the development of effective multidisciplinary and collaborative models of care.

There was a marked degree of consensus amongst those involved in the study, suggesting a strong link between vulnerability to HIV transmission in children and young people and their socio-economic status. This suggests that policies for children and prevention strategies need to embrace a more holistic approach which *recognises* this interaction between social deprivation factors and good health.

The questionnaire

A questionnaire was circulated to all National Children's Bureau members as part of an information gathering exercise for the report. The main purpose of the questionnaire was to get some idea, however impressionistic, of the problems, issues and concerns which agencies were currently experiencing, and to give respondents an opportunity to comment on aspects of service developments, needs and gaps. The questionnaire was circulated to National Children's Bureau members which included local authorities in England, Wales and Scotland, and Northern Ireland Boards; district health authorities; voluntary organisations; educational bodies; government departments; professional associations; and National Children's Bureau groups. Agencies were invited to include any relevant materials or documentation if they wished, and were given a time limit for response (*see* Appendix 1 for a sample copy of the questionnaire). Time did not allow for the piloting of the questionnaire and, in hindsight, some questions could have been more appropriately phrased to elicit more appropriate answers.

The response rate was very encouraging and has provided an important and useful channel of communication for diverse organisations who have welcomed the National Children's Bureau's initiative. Many respondents commented positively on the opportunity it created for them to express their views and concerns. For some organisations it has clearly acted as a catalyst in promoting further internal reviews concerning on-going programmes or identifying issues for clarification and development.

The true response rate was actually much higher than the total number of returned completed questionnaires (146). Many agencies preferred to comment by letter and supplied copies of agency publications, materials and policy guidelines, including a wide range of health education and prevention materials. Some wanted in particular to comment on specific areas of concern.

Table 1.1 gives details of types and numbers of agencies which completed and returned questionnaires. The detailed questionnaire analysis appears in Appendix 2.

Table 1.1 Completed questionnaires

Breakdown by agency	Numbers	%
Health authorities	59	40.4
Social service department	33	22.6
Voluntary organisations	31	21.3
Education authorities	14	9.5
Others	9	6.2
Total	146	

Forty per cent of all replies came from medical staff in health care settings and 43 per cent were from voluntary and social services. Only nine per cent of Local Education Authorities responded, although they are the most likely after District Health Authorities to have direct involvement with children and young people with HIV, as the majority of children with HIV are in the school population. The cumulative total number of infected children aged 14 years or less with HIV (including those with haemophilia) for the UK as of 30 September 1990 were 407.[2] The total number of AIDS cases were 49.

Part II
Discussion of issues in relation to HIV and AIDS

2. Making sense of the data on children with HIV and AIDS

The presentation of HIV and AIDS statistics for children can be misleading about the actual number of children with HIV infection in the child population and this is unhelpful and hinders a realistic assessment of needs for planning services. It is worrying that despite predictions of increased HIV infection in women of child bearing age, until recently there has been limited speculation about the impact this will have on child numbers. The absence of debate has possibly led to a falsely optimistic view that infectivity in children is statistically so insignificant (less than one per cent according to The Cox Report[3]), that there is little cause for concern or need for proactive planning. This false complacency does a disservice to children who are infected now, and who are not able to make their needs known or to alert policy makers about the problems and difficulties they face.

Ascertaining the actual numbers of children with HIV infection and AIDS in the UK – by age group, geographical distribution and needs – from the published data is both confusing and misleading. The Communicable Disease Surveyance Centre (CDSC) report focuses on only one exposure category for children infected, that is, children considered to be at risk of HIV who are born to a woman who is HIV positive. However, it lists the following exposure categories:

- homosexual/bisexual males;
- injecting drug user;
- heterosexual contact;
- haemophilia and blood/components recipients;
- children of at-risk/infected parent;
- other/undetermined.

Whilst it is acknowledged that estimating future patterns of infection in children is closely related to the number of infected women of child bearing age, it is not the *only* factor. Children who acquire HIV infection sexually or by injecting drug use are not identified. Haemophilia children with HIV infection are not expected to increase in numbers following effective treatment of Factor VIII blood products, but this is still significantly the largest single category of children currently infected. However, in official returns children are subsumed into the exposure category for all haemophiliacs. A further confusion arises if it is not understood that, statistically, children are defined as those of 14 years or under. This definition excludes significant numbers of infected children in the 15–19-year-old age group who are in need. Determining patterns of distribution for children is also difficult except in the exposure category of children born to women who are HIV positive, where significant clusters of these 'at risk' children have been identified in Edinburgh and the four Thames Regions in London. Reporting numbers of children by District Health Authorities is further obscured as numbers of less than ten in any one exposure category are not given – supposedly based on the need to protect confidentiality in areas of low numbers. However, this under-reporting leads to false assumptions by agencies involved in service provision that there is no need for forward planning.

Recently commissioned work on forecasting future costs and care planning on HIV/AIDS services in two of the leading London districts makes little mention of future care planning for children.[4] One report rationalises this based on lack of quantative experience. Yet both districts are already providing services for HIV positive women and some children, through STD clinics, drug services, antenatal clinics and paediatric departments. Making connections between the needs of HIV positive women and possible future increases in child numbers is acknowledged but, as yet, has not led to articulate policies and plans for children. It is acknowledged that the numbers of women and children who are HIV infected is likely to be an underestimate. Because most testing is performed on a voluntary basis, many will be unaware of their HIV status – and may not wish to know. Pregnant women are now offered the HIV test in ante-natal clinics and, consequently, they may be over-represented in the population.

Given the difficulties of forecasting future numbers of infected children the recent PHLS report in January 1990 for England, Wales and Ireland, suggested a range of 'no more than 300 children at the end of 1988 . . . and (this) might rise to 500 at the end of 1990 as an upper limit'. This referred only to the exposure category of children of an at-risk/infected parent. (In 1990, approximately 100 of these children were less than one year of age and it is necessary to wait until chidren reach 18 months to 2 years before maternal anti-body is lost and infection status is determined.) Up to December 1989 there were 23 AIDS deaths reported in children born to an HIV positive parent. Thus an opportunity to inform the public about the overall numbers of children possibly infected from all routes of transmission was not addressed. Ironically, in 1987 expert witnesses to the Social Services Committee on Problems Associated with AIDS were already sounding the alarm bells about adults when the number of reported AIDS cases diagnosed was approximately 610, and HIV infection cases approximately 3877.[5] By December 1989 there were 1,251 HIV positive females of whom 1,027 were in the age group 15–44-years-old.

Estimating numbers of children currently infected *is* difficult, but greater clarity in presenting information on known cases would at least encourage a more open and honest debate. By separating children into different exposure categories, the overall figure is fragmented and assumptions that very few children are infected are reinforced. If the numbers of haemophiliac children of 15–19 years (126) who are HIV positive are added to the number of children under 14 years from the two other exposure categories, the cumulative total figure of 895 HIV infected children is arrived at (ranging in age from 0–19 years) living in the UK.[6] As this is likely to be an underestimate, it is surely time to recognise that, in the words of the Social Services Committee's 7th Report on AIDS, 'there is a need for more intensive research so that figures can be obtained on which to plan'.[7]

A recent study of anonymous testing of neonates in the Thames Region (using the Guthrie test) found that although HIV positive rates were relatively low, there was an indication that six children in every 100,000 tested revealed the presence of maternal HIV anti-body positive status. On closer analysis, rates for Inner London were 0.49 per cent compared with 0.04 per cent for Outer London.[8] The planned large scale anonymous screening surveillance programmes for newborn babies and pregnant women at sentinel, STD and Drug Dependency clinics may provide more accurate forecasting in the future, but at present, with heterosexual infection increasing, it should be assumed that there are more children infected with HIV than have been currently reported. From April 1991 the British Paediatric Surveillance Unit will be responsible for publishing regular bulletins on HIV infection in the UK and Irish Republic.[9]

Ethnic monitoring statistics are not yet reported. However, this study revealed that some agencies are hindered in developing ethnically-sensitive services because families and children with HIV infection have been reluctant to disclose their HIV status and seek help. Meeting diverse multiracial needs can only be honestly addressed if better information is collated and made available to aid the planning of services.

The PHLS Communicable Disease Surveillance Centre (CDSC) intends to change the presention of HIV/AIDS statistics from January 1991 which will emphasise the probable routes of infection rather than exposure categories (*see* Appendix 4).[10] A recent re-examination of the presentation of HIV/AIDS statistics by Clive Stevens has suggested a different approach which provides separate columns for children by age, sex and risk behaviour (*see* Appendix 3).[11] The London Borough of Hammersmith and Fulham Social Services Department HIV Unit is collating data on numbers of affected children by age, sex, ethnic origin, disability, HIV status – well or unwell, and location. This enables services for children to be monitored and developed according to *client needs*. Individual care plans are costed, and service managers are rebated according to what services the client uses. Through the joint care planning mechanisms, guidance on services and good practice for children with HIV/AIDS has also been agreed, covering all aspects of care – from antenatal services to services in the schools and community.

Recommendations

Research should be commissioned on the possibilities of refining present collation and dissemination of data on children – exploring different models and approaches. The following areas should be examined and information presented.

Probable routes of infection

For example:

- children at risk from infected parent;
- blood/blood products;
- sexual transmission;
- injecting drug use;
- multiple risks;
- other;
- insufficient information.

Age breakdown 0–18 years

- 0–3
- 3–5
- 5–10
- 10–14
- 14–18+

Special needs

For example:

- haemophilia;
- disabilities;
- educational;
- ethnicity;
- HIV impairment;
  – well – asymptomatic
  – symptomatic
  – AIDS;
- drug use.

Social indicators

For example:

- housing accommodation;
- income levels;
- single parents;
- family size;
- family profile
  – own parents
  – fostered/adopted
  – in care.

Geographical distribution in the UK

For example:

- NHS Regions and Districts;
- Local Authorities.

3. Womens issues –
a disease of the family

This chapter is concerned with reviewing the complexity of HIV related issues and the impact on women within the context of family relationships and social roles.

The number of women infected with HIV is increasing world-wide. Women in the USA now account for 9 per cent and in Europe for 13 per cent of reported AIDS cases. AIDS is the leading cause of death among women aged 25–40 years in New York City, where between 35,000–40,000 women of child-bearing age are now infected with HIV. These women are mainly from Black and Hispanic communities.[12]

In the UK up to December 1989, 1,251 women had been infected – of these approximately 45 per cent were injecting drug users and 30 per cent had acquired the virus heterosexually. Heterosexual spread of the virus is increasing but predictions remain uncertain about the rate at which this will happen. The pattern of HIV infection in women in Britain varies, with a higher proportion of women infected residing in Scotland – 25 per cent compared to 7 per cent in the rest of the UK. Most of these women, like their counterparts in Europe, USA and the Third World, are young women of 15–44 years of age, capable of child bearing. By implication, it is from this group of infected women that children at risk of HIV vertical transmission will be born. Public concern is centred on whether this rise in the number of young infected women will be mirrored by a similar rise in the number of newly infected babies. Up to now, research has suggested that one in four babies are likely to be infected and women who are already ill may have a higher transmission rate but a recent study has revised infectivity rates downwards to 13 per cent.[13] In response to this concern public policies have tended to concentrate on HIV ante-natal screening procedures, even though there is evidence of a high refusal rate by women when offered the choice of a test, because of the level of fear, anxiety and stigmatisation associated with the test. Despite these anxieties felt by women faced with an HIV test, one study of screening procedures found that few units had access to a trained counsellor. The study went on to suggest that clear policies on patient consent and counselling are essential, before *any* testing strategy is implemented.[14]

Some health workers have agreed that any strategy for preventing mother to child transmission must focus more on the needs of women in terms of their own risks and well-being. It is therefore crucial that the needs of *all* women are addressed in relation to the impact of HIV.

Many women will be affected by HIV. They may be infected themselves or living in families where partners and children are infected – for example, families affected by haemophilia. They may be ill themselves but acting as carers for other sick members of the family. They may be carers in their professional lives in services such as childcare, social work, teaching and health care, and they may perform important health educational roles, both in public services and/or informally as carers in the community. The major burden of caring may well fall on *informal carers* who will need good local support systems and a network of out-reach services to counteract social isolation and deprivation.

All women will need to be aware of HIV transmission and how to protect themselves. They will need access to comprehensive services covering contraceptive and reproductive advice, health promotion, safer sex and drug use, counselling on HIV testing and access to pregnancy advice – including abortion and bereavement counselling, and good ante-natal and post-natal care. They will also need information on caring for HIV infected children, knowledge about services such as welfare benefits, housing, legal advice and how to stay healthy.

Agonising choices may confront a woman and her partner about having children. Counselling on pregnancy requires expert knowledge and advisory skills. A woman and her partner need to understand *all* the risks before making a decision – the risk to the potential mother, her partner and her unborn child. Some women living with an infected partner may wish to risk transmission if it means having the child of a beloved person who may die. A woman, married to a young haemophiliac with HIV, made this decision after considering the risk to herself and her child. In another situation a woman with HIV infection, who was already showing symptoms of HIV, decided to proceed with her pregnancy because she had longed for a child and has subsequently made plans with her family for the care of her child after her death.

In a study of women with HIV attending an ante-natal clinic, most women decided to continue with their pregnancies even when early abortion was offered. This confirms similar findings of studies of women's attitudes towards their pregnancies carried out in the USA. Many women, particularly those from disadvantaged groups, see motherhood as an important and positive act, giving them a sense of purpose and self respect. Many seek help at this time in changing their behaviour (if they are misusing drugs), taking greater responsibility and care of themselves in preparing for motherhood.

Information on ascertaining the risk factors which may accelerate HIV infection in adults and children is, as yet, inconclusive. Early studies suggest that risk transmission from an HIV infected mother to her unborn child increases if the mother is already showing significant symptoms of HIV disease, and therefore women may choose to have their babies in the earlier stages of HIV disease rather than later. It is thought that pregnancy itself does not worsen the prognosis for a mother's health, unless she has AIDS, when maternal health may be worse. In a study of obstetric outcome of low birth weight babies in Edinburgh, the HIV status of the mother was found to be of less significance than other factors such as social deprivation, smoking, unemployment, drug use, late presentation in pregnancy, or being an unsupported parent.[16]

In weighing up decisions about pregnancy and procreation, all HIV positive women will need access to expert advice and counselling which should be tailored to individual needs and risk factors. A study based on the experience of counselling 92 HIV positive pregnant women identified six points in reaching a decision:[17]

1 Fact finding

- establishing circumstances of pregnancy, the desire for a child and the mother's health and HIV status;
- drug use, sexuality, relationships;
- existence of support networks, access to services and back-up.

2 *Options*

- whether to conceive or not;
- whether to terminate or not;
- consider alternatives such as adoption, fostering, egg, sperm or embryo donation;
- examining their own and their partner's feelings and needs.

3 *Decision-making*

- looking at the *process* of decision making in the short term – which may help towards reaching decisions over long term goals.

4 *Living with the consequences*

- consider how to handle the decision – sometimes compromises will have to be made.

5 *Consider practical assistance*

- social services;
- finance;
- support;
- respite care;
- information;
- help lines;
- telephone.

6 *Continued support*

- consider the long term problems such as coping with uncertainty, loss and separation;
- consider the practical and emotional difficulties of caring for a sick child, coupled with feelings of guilt, low self-esteem and feeling responsible.

Women from Black and minority ethnic communities may be especially isolated and vulnerable, and services need to be aware of the importance of providing information in minority languages. Interpreters and link workers will also be needed who can liaise with significant local community leaders from different ethnic, religious and cultural communities.

Until recently there were few organisations catering specifically for the needs of women. Positively Women was established to offer emotional and practical support, advice and counselling on coping with the problems of living with HIV infection. Over 500 women have been in contact with the organisation, and 50 per cent of these women have children. Their experience has led them to believe that there are many women with HIV who are still not known to anyone. They often face medical ignorance and inadequate treatment, even after diagnosis. For example, GPs often fail to realise that a woman with the virus should have a cervical test six-monthly because of the increased risk of cervical cancer. These women need help and advice with medical care and treatment for themselves and their children. They need access to legal and welfare services, and they need re-housing.

Women with HIV who have children often face tremendous problems with housing, and have great difficulty in getting re-housed. In Scotland, the need to help women with HIV was identified earlier, perhaps because the number of *known* HIV cases is higher there. Many women in Scotland have acquired HIV through injecting drug use, and have children who are also infected. The Aberlour Trust established Brenda House, a housing project which provides living accommodation (six flats) for women with HIV and their children. The project aims to support women in caring for themselves and their children, and offers intensive support in drug rehabilitation and preparation for independent living. Some of the experiences of women in Brenda House are described (*see* Chapter 16) to illustrate the importance of listening to those who speak directly from their experience and by doing so expose the gulf that separates service providers from those who use them.

The major group of women infected with HIV are those who are associated with injecting drug use or are the sexual partner of a drug user. Most women affected are likely to have low socio-economic status and fragmented family relationships. They are often single parents, living in poverty and poor housing. In addition, they may have experienced violent and abusing relationships and may hold anti-authoritarian attitudes. As individuals, they often have a poor self image, low self-esteem and will suffer from guilt, self-hate and disapproval – and may be reluctant to seek help, fearing the social stigma of HIV infection and *further* rejection.[18]

Other women affected by HIV may be living in very different family situations, and planners need to be aware of these family patterns when planning services (*see* Chapter 4, Family profiles). A common fear is that their children may be taken into care if their HIV status is revealed, and this feeling may be reinforced by attitudes towards drug misusing parents – which make assumptions that they are, automatically, inadequate parents. Although this assumption is often challenged by experienced drug workers who work with drug using families, it can be difficult to counteract prejudicial attitudes.

Comparisons are often drawn between the pattern of HIV infection in women in New York City and Edinburgh, leading to speculation and fears of a similar explosion of infectivity rates among disadvantaged women, and a consequent rise in the number of infected children. Although these fears cannot be dismissed, they need to be treated with some caution. Although both groups of women come from similar disadvantaged backgrounds, there are some important differences, and equally important lessons to be learned from them. In the USA, the Alan Guttmacher Institute's comparative study of developed countries (including the UK) investigated the contraceptive behaviour of adolescents.[19] It found that US teenagers have much lower rates of contraceptive use and much higher rates of child bearing, abortion and pregnancy than those found in other developed countries – even though the level of adolescent sexuality appeared to be quite similar in all the countries studied. Explanations for these differences suggest that in countries other than the USA, contraceptive care was more likely to be integrated into primary health services, available at convenient times and localities, and offered either free or at a low cost to everyone. There was also greater dissemination of information in schools and a greater involvement of pharmacists in the distribution of literature.

The alarming increase in children with HIV infection born to mainly Black and Hispanic women in urban populations such as New York City, Boston and New Jersey, reflects the higher rates of pregnancy in this group compared to white women. In the USA pregnancy rates for Black women are twice that of white women, and over 40 per cent of Black women have their first child in their teens, and four out of five are born outside marriage. These women are less likely to have access to early ante-natal care and more likely to give birth to low weight babies. Twice as many babies from this group are likely to die in the first year of life than in their white counterparts, and over 25 per cent are born with a health problem. These women are also less likely to have any form of medical insurance and, although Medicaid is available free to pregnant women; different states apply differing criteria for claiming benefits.

In the UK, in comparison, it is interesting to note that there has been a rise in contraceptive take-up of 13–15-year-olds attending family planning clinics and research suggests that the increase in sexual activity for under 16-year-olds is not reflected in an increased number of conceptions (including births and abortions). However, it also cautions that although there is evidence that young people are becoming more effective users of contraception, there are 12 per cent of sexually active 16-year-olds who have never used any form of birth control. It is therefore a cause for concern that a recent survey by the Family Planning Association reported widespread *cuts* in family planning clinic services – with one in four sessions lost.[20] Yet these clinics are exceptionally well-used and the preferred choice for young women seeking advice on contraception, sexuality and sex education. There is a fear that this reduction in services will lead to increased abortion rates and unwanted pregnancies.

One worrying trend that mirrors the experience of Black and Hispanic women in the USA is the poorer outcome in the UK in perinatal rates for children born to teenage mothers and the increasing class differential which adversely affects the children born to the poorest women in British society. (Reported by OPCS Mortality Statistics *Review of the Registrar General on deaths in England and Wales 1987*, table two.)

A recent report from Edinburgh has suggested that there is evidence of a silent HIV epidemic among heterosexuals between 15–40 years of age, affecting one in every 100 men and one in 250 women.[21] Of the 16 new cases reporting heterosexual transmission, 12 were women – some of whom may have been infected after only one episode of heterosexual intercourse.

If lessons are to be learnt from the US experience it would suggest that the most important weapon in fighting HIV transmission is to increase the access, use and take-up of primary health care and education programmes in deprived communities, and to strengthen the links between the welfare infra-structure, within a free, fully funded National Health Service. Perhaps the most effective protection for disadvantaged women and their children is to be found by focusing on their needs for well-integrated locally-based services which are friendly, non-judgemental and accessible – and to provide secure housing and financial support as a foundation upon which to build. (See recommendations at the end of this Chapter.)

Living with HIV – 'Why don't you ask us what we think?'

This section gives a brief account of a discussion held with a group of women whose lives have been deeply affected by HIV and, using their words, gives an insight into their experiences.

On HIV Testing

'I did not realise I had been tested for HIV until someone told me in the most casual and brutal way that I was positive. Perhaps they felt it didn't matter how they treated me because I was a drug user and I'm not worth bothering with.'

'I think it's very important where you go to have the test and who does it. I don't really understand what is meant by "pre-test counselling" – I certainly didn't have any explanation. I think you should be given proper written information beforehand, so that you can think about it before you decide. It's also important to take someone with you, a friend or someone you trust. It's important not to be alone when you get your results of the test.'

'When I was told I was HIV positive my first reaction was one of total disbelief and shock, followed by awful depression. I felt quite numb inside, and didn't leave the house for a month. I wouldn't tell anyone, not even my family or friends. I was very frightened that once the neighbours and my friends knew, they would have nothing to do with me or my children. I didn't want anyone to know for the sake of protecting the children – I didn't want them to suffer. I was worried that the other kids would be nasty to them and refuse to play with them.'

On having a baby

'I was put in a separate room when I was in labour. The nurses wouldn't come near me, and treated me like a leper. I was frightened and left alone. There was a notice on the door warning other staff to keep out. No other patients came near me after the baby was born, and the staff all wore gowns and masks whenever they picked up the baby. Do you think a woman who has just had a spina bifida baby would have been treated in the same way? Why should they treat her with sympathy, but me with such disrespect?'

'I wasn't allowed to use the bathroom until the nurse had disinfected it.

Some of the staff were incredibly discriminatory and over-reacted when I was admitted as an emergency. Their reaction was almost hysterical – I couldn't believe it.'

'I was refused admission to my local and nearest hospital when the doctor told them I was HIV positive, even though I was dangerously ill and haemorrhaging. I was finally admitted to a hospital about 20 miles away.'

Living with HIV

'The psychological problems of trying to live with the fact that you are HIV is terrible – or worrying that you might be, or that your child might be positive.'

'I dread the days I have to go to the hospital to have the baby tested again. I have to screw my courage up to go, it's agony waiting for the results of the test – even when the result is negative, the relief is tinged with fear and anxiety, because you know it's not finished with. You still have to keep going back. This will go on for a long time until they are sure that he's clear.'

'I never go alone to the clinic, its important to have someone with you to give you emotional support. I dread going.'

'I didn't know I was HIV until my husband died. He was a drug addict and I went to the hospital to collect his clothes. They told me he had AIDS and I had better get a test. I was terribly angry at the way they treated me – they made me feel completely worthless. Coping with the grief, shock and bereavement of losing my husband has been shattering, but I have to stay as fit and as well as possible for the sake of my children. I find it difficult to talk to them about my illness. Sometimes they ask me if I'm going to die – and I don't know what to say to them.'

'I've got one brother who has died of AIDS and another relative who has AIDS – he's married to my cousin. I think she'd fall apart if she didn't have lots of support from the women's group and being able to come here everyday and leave her little girls in the playgroup. Although they have both been tested and are negative it doesn't seem to make any difference. It's terrible to live with the knowledge that your husband is going to die – and you keep wondering if you really are in the clear.'

'I was determined to come off drugs because I really wanted to have this baby. Having the baby was the best decision I ever made. I've been drug free for over a year, and so far the baby's making good progress. I've got HIV but I'm going to stay well so that I can see my daughter grow up. We spend a lot of time trying to claim the right amount of welfare benefits. It's difficult explaining what your needs are when you've got HIV. We've had our benefits cut off often without any explanation – nobody seems to understand that it costs more when you are on a special diet.'

'It's not easy to try to kick your drug habit; it's important to keep regularly in touch with the Community Psychiatric Nurse. If people are to try to reduce their drug intake and go through a rehabilitation programme they need intensive support from the health visitor, CPN, and out-reach workers. We all know people on drugs who need help but won't go near social services or a voluntary agency. Out-reach workers can sometimes befriend women who really are quite frightened and hopefully gain their confidence, and help them if they want to change their drug habit.'

'We still think that most information you read about HIV is not written in simple enough language that ordinary people understand. We should all have better information. Before people start telling us what's good for us and what we need, they should actually ask us what *we* think. We *know*, because we live with HIV – it's us and our kids who are getting sick.'

'Before a housing project like this is set up, it's important to talk to other residents and local tenants' associations about their reactions and views. Many people had all kinds of distorted ideas about AIDS, and at our first public meeting local people were against the idea of the project. There were people there who thought they would catch AIDS just by walking in the same street! They were worried about our kids playing with their kids. It took a lot of careful preparation, work and education – explaining what the project aimed to do, asking for their help and support and careful health education – so that people really had an opportunity to understand how difficult it is to get HIV disease unless you practice risky behaviour. Gradually we won local people over. Other neighbours, instead of denying problems, started to acknowledge that they too had a son, friend or relative who had a drug or alcohol problem or knew 'someone' who had the virus. It's still not easy; it will take time for people to realise that we're just ordinary people who want to do the best we can for our families and live a normal life in the community.'

'I feel safe when I come here to the centre; I don't have to pretend all the time. At least I can share my feelings with others – I know they'll understand because we're all scared sometimes about what's going to happen to us or our children.'

'I know the children worry a lot, and so does my husband. Fathers need to grieve and talk about their feelings, but they find it very difficult. He won't discuss making plans for the children if anything happens to us – I know my mum will look after them. But some couples don't have anyone they can turn to – but I know they don't want the kids to go into care.'

What we would like to change

'First of all, we want to be treated like human beings with respect and dignity. We have met great kindness from lots of staff in the hospitals, but we have also had appalling treatment, and confidential information has been given out to people without permission.'

'We think all hospital staff should have proper training about HIV/AIDS. Some of the staff were very ignorant – it's not fair to expose sick people to these ignorant attitudes. No one should be allowed to work in the hospital unless they are prepared to handle and care for all types of cases. This includes the porters and ward cleaners as well as doctors and nurses.'

'Doctors still find it very difficult to explain to the patient what's involved with their treatment and diagnosis. They don't tell you anything. They should be prepared to listen to our worries and problems – I often worry because I don't really understand what the drugs are for. It would help if we were given better medical information and kept our own medical record cards, so that we could check back afterwards on what medicine we are taking and can ask questions. We do want to know what children can or can't do when they've got HIV. It's important when you've got HIV to be able to talk to your children and prepare them for what may happen. It's important to have support for parents and children from skilled workers, like health visitors and project staff, so if we're upset and worried we know we've got people to help us – especially when we get very depressed. It's important to have on-going support from care staff for both parents and children.'

'We think housing accommodation with lots of support is very important. There are times when we go through an awful crisis. Lots of things can trigger it off and, at times like that, you can hold on if there are people around to support you, and know what you're going through.'

Recommendations

Health and local authorities, voluntary organisations and user groups should collaborate in drawing up comprehensive HIV/AIDS policies and strategies for women and children, with guidance on what constitutes good practice. Plans should be published and information about services widely disseminated to local communities and women's groups. Services should include provision of the following:

- Family Planning Clinics;
- Well Woman Clinics;
- Drug Dependency Clinics;
- Needle Exchange Schemes;
- Street Agencies;
- Out-reach Health Prevention Programmes;
- Drug Rehabilitation Services;
- Housing Accommodation;
- Drop-in Centres;
- Creches, Nurseries, Daily minders, Playgroups;
- Respite Care;
- Home Care;
- Fostering and Adoption Services;
- Residential Care.

Maternity and Health Care Services should have agreed policies and procedures on:

- HIV testing;
- HIV counselling and support;
- integrated infection control procedures which are non-discriminatory and apply to all women;
- ante-natal and post-natal care offering a continuum of treatment from hospital to the Community;
- confidentiality and record keeping;
- separate abortion and bereavement counselling;
- 'shared care' between hospital departments such as obstetrics, gynaecology and paediatrics;
- the relationship between paediatric hospital care and community paediatrics, including the role of the health visitor and general practitioner;
- care plans for mother and child – which may involve support for drug dependency or maintenance, with support for withdrawal;
- encouraging women to understand and be fully consulted about their treatments plans – including monitoring their health and their child's;

- giving advice on nutrition, diet and preventative health measures such as stress reduction. This advice should be made available as part of a holistic approach to maintaining positive health;
- reaching women who's first language is not English. They should have access to professionally trained health workers who can act as interpreters and advocates. Religious and cultural differences in respect of childcare practice should be acknowledged and respected.

4. Family profiles

Families living with HIV disease – what are their needs?

Reports from OPCS surveys show that families living with children with disabilities are likely to suffer more from emotional and psychological stresses (such as depression, insomnia, fatigue and anxiety) than other families.[22] They are likely to have poor general health, lower incomes and a higher dependence on state benefits, with three quarters of single parent families dependent on state benefits as a main source of income. Despite lack of respite care, adequate transport services, and so on, the majority of children live with their own families. Only a minority are placed in residential care, usually as a consequence of overriding social problems, rather than because of their disability.

Remarkably similar characteristics are also seen in families living with HIV. Most children with HIV are still living at home with their own parents and, in common with other disabilities, often suffer multiple social deprivation and have high social needs for better support systems. A minority of children have been placed in foster care or adopted, usually because of problems related to family disfunction rather than to the HIV status of the child.

Despite these similarities it is apparent that families with HIV have additional and complex burdens to carry which impact powerfully on the whole family system, placing great strain on the capacity of families to cope with social and personal distress. These burdens include the devastating impact of living with an incurable, and potentially fatal, stigmatising disease. Added to this is the guilt and blame associated or apportioned between family members – who is 'at fault' – relating to transmission of the virus within the family. Infected injecting drug using parents or other partners who have acquired the virus through their own risky behaviour, may be consumed with guilt, remorse, grief and blame at transmitting the virus to a child or partner. Grandparents have to confront the painful knowledge that their children and grandchildren may well die before they do, and some may have to take over parental care when they are becoming frail and less able to take the physical strain of parenting. Parents may face difficulties in acknowledging their own possible death before their children reach adulthood, and will need to make plans for the surviving children to be cared for by other family members, friends or professional carers.

Secrecy is an instinctive protective response from many parents. They keep the knowledge of their own or their children's HIV status from the children to protect them from the pain of social ostracism and prejudicial reactions of neighbours, other relatives, or the school. In doing so they may reinforce paranoid behaviour and secrecy. Families may withdraw from everyday social contacts, fearing exposure, and turn in upon themselves. Denial of any problem may be a marked feature, influencing all members of the family to be part of the conspiracy of silence. When this occurs, strong emotional feelings concerning their grief, anger and fears about death and dying cannot be acknowledged – making it more difficult for families to come to terms with their own sadness and loss, or to create opportunities to express feelings of love and affection for each other. Sexual problems and marital difficulties can also be exacerbated because partners are living with such high levels of stress and anxiety.

Financial hardship will be an increasing burden for some families where there is multiple ill health, since the additional costs of illness such as special diets, transportation or hospital visits are multiplied within one family unit. Payments for child minding and relief care, loss of earnings or unemployment – resulting from illness can all have a devastating effect on the life of the family.

Maintaining family well-being and strengths in combating HIV disease is an important goal in service planning, and is more likely to be achieved if families are offered a continuum of care which provides a 'seamless' service for children and families which transcends service boundaries. Providing individual care packages to suit differing family needs is the preferred option, provided that families are supported in their choices and are seen as full partners in decision-making and as sharing power with the professionals.

Although all families have universal needs for access to good care this can only be achieved if services are specifically targeted to reach groups who may, for many reasons, have unequal access to services. To achieve this, the reasons why certain groups suffer inequality of access to services must be identified and countered. This study identified six broadly based family categories and their characteristics, which will influence how services for children and their families with differing needs are met. These categories of need are discussed in the following six sections.

Stigmatised families

The stigmatised family with HIV disease would conform closely to some of the families in Edinburgh whose family profiles include strong associations with injecting drug use as a major factor in HIV transmission, allied with multiple social deprivation. Families usually live in the same neighbourhood and develop their own networks and sub-culture based on their drug habit. This sets them apart from other neighbours and reinforces social ostracism. However, within the drug culture they gain support from others who share similar experiences of stigma.

Stigmatised families will usually have experienced services as judgemental, punitive and unsympathetic. Consequently, they will be reluctant to seek help until a crisis erupts, fearing rejection or policies which criminalise their drug habit and threaten family unity by taking children into care – sometimes with very little evidence of bad parenting. Breaking down barriers of distrust and alienation are crucial if families stigmatised by HIV infection are to receive appropriate help and support. Families have to be *convinced* that services are open, non-judgemental and accessible.

Work pioneered in Edinburgh in working with stigmatised families suggests that, despite previous perceptions, families can be helped when offered intensive, locally targeted services which meet the expressed desire for families to continue to care for their HIV children – even when parents themselves may be quite ill with HIV disease. The majority of children infected with HIV have remained with their parents or relatives, and have only been received into care when other factors related to broader social problems of family breakdown have occurred. Probably because there is a large local population of drug users in Edinburgh it has perhaps been easier to galvanise all three services of health, education and social services into looking imaginatively at a broad range of provision. However, it may be difficult to replicate this range of provision and resources elsewhere, where it is less easy to identify significant numbers of stigmatised drug related families in one locality.

In Edinburgh, services for women and children have been pioneered by a voluntary childcare agency, the Aberlour Child Care Trust. The Trust offers intensive residential rehabilitation drug programmes which combine childcare arrangements, family support and therapy with hospital – and community – based paediatric and primary health care services. Support and counselling for mothers and liaison with drug services, including community psychiatric nurses, takes place. Long term care planning for children who may face the loss of a sick parent is organised when parents wish arrangements to be made. Help with moving back into less supported accommodation is the objective, although with long term needs of sick parents and children, the necessity for longer-term transitional accommodation, respite provision, and hospice care is becoming more apparent. A programme of community education about HIV and drug related issues was an essential preparatory initiative in gaining support and recognition for the project work, and in allaying fears and myths about families who misuse drugs and HIV disease.

The community paediatric team based in the local hospital has developed comprehensive health care monitoring and treatment for HIV infected children and their parents. Children are regularly monitored and followed up in community clinics and home visits are made by hospital staff. Families are also offered on-going access at times of crisis and emergency. Individual members of a family often need to meet separately with professionals and talk about the problems of managing their child's illness, diet, medication, and so on. Links are also made by the community paediatrician with head teachers and schools, so that support can be offered to teachers who may be worried about a particular child within the school population. Schools are, it must be noted, concerned to maintain information about a child's HIV status as confidential.

Working with families affected by HIV infection who have a drug related problem can mean acknowledging the complexity of inter-generational family relationships and conflicts. For example, in one family a mother, father, and three of their four children were HIV infected. The oldest (uninfected) child's needs were ignored and forgotten because of the medical and social needs of the others. Siblings are often unable to discuss what is happening in the family and may feel very frightened and isolated – becoming non-communicative and depressed. This child was in her early teens and needed help in looking at her future bereavement. There is, clearly, a need to provide sensitive counselling and bereavement services for children and young individuals who may be presented with powerful negative images which associate sexuality, drug misuse and death with HIV disease.

In another situation, a grandmother was caring for her five-year-old grandchild (who was HIV positive) because her daughter was terminally ill with AIDS. The grandmother refused to allow the child to visit her mother and, when she died, was unable to talk to her grandchild about her mother's death.

There is, undoubtedly, an increasing need to provide hospice care for women and children, and transitional group homes where a terminally sick parent, who may also be dependent on drugs, and wishes to continue to care for her children can do so. It is often wrongly assumed that fathers in drug related HIV families may well be absent or disinterested, but this is not always the case. Sometimes they are in prison or on probation, and close liaison is necessary for supporting and counselling absentee fathers through the probation and prison service. Fathers may be very involved in caring for children, but may feel consumed with guilt if they have transmitted the HIV virus to their wife and child because of their drug habits. Family counselling for *all* members may be essential, and men, in particular, may need additional support in helping them to acknowl-edge feelings of grief, loss and guilt. This is especially true in cultures where it is not generally acceptable for men to express their emotions (except at ritual events such as football matches where to hug, cry and kiss each other is allowed).

In conclusion, some of the approaches pioneered in Edinburgh, in working with stigmatised families should be replicated elsewhere. This will, however, require intensive and coordinated support from all agencies, and should include provision of good childcare services, supported accommodation, family counselling, and drug mainte-nance and rehabilitation programmes.

Isolated families and families from Black and minority ethnic groups

Some evidence has arisen out of this study which suggests that there are growing numbers of children and families with HIV who are more socially isolated than others because of certain factors which inhibit them from gaining access to appropriate help and support. These are likely to be families who live in smaller communities and towns, or inner cities, and families from Black and minority ethnic communities who have come from overseas to work or study in the UK.

The first group, those living in small communities, are reluctant to reveal their HIV status because of fears of ostracism from, and rejection by, other members of the community. They may also live some distance from major treatment centres and have few opportunities to share common concerns with other families or experienced health care staff who can advise them professionally. Not all families will feel sufficiently resourceful or emotionally tough enough to challenge local prejudices or stigma. Families that have done so have usually been substitute families – foster parents or adopters – with a great deal of back-up and support from social services and paediatric staff in campaigning to change attitudes of local parents at schools and playgroups. Families where a child and parents may be unwell may prefer to make contact with national organisations such as Positively Women or the Terrence Higgins Trust for counselling and support. Telephone advice and counselling can be helpful and this is sometimes the preferred way of seeking help rather than taking the risk of confiding in local family and friends.

The difficulties of parents who are distant from experienced treatment centres do concern them, and some have persuaded their doctor to refer them to tertiary centres for treatment and have established links between the local hospital and the paediatric hospital for shared care of patients. For isolated families who wish to retain a low profile, there is a need to develop better information and resources which can be made available locally. For example, if local joint strategies for HIV services and policies have been agreed, there should be an information and resource centre in every locality where confidential advice, support and counselling can be offered. The Body Positive Women's Group has established volunteer support groups for women with children and tries to link up isolated families with volunteers who live near them. The Group also runs regular drop-in meetings at weekends for those who may prefer to travel away from their home town.

There are a significant number of families from overseas who are less likely to present for care and treatment early on in their illness because of overcoming religious, cultural, and language barriers – and racism. Problems related to HIV infection in this group often only come to the attention of medical and care staff when a child or parent is already quite ill and a family crisis erupts.

Complex issues have to be faced in working with different family belief systems and cultures. For example, a Muslim father found it difficult to accept help from a female social worker because of his pride and his belief that it showed weakness to be helped by a woman. Efforts must be made to understand and respect cultural differences if minority ethnic families with HIV are to be effectively helped. Several reasons have been put forward to explain why families from Black and minority ethnic communities are reluctant to seek help, and these are discussed in Chapter 12 on *Black and minority ethnic issues*. The chapter also makes recommendations for developing ethnically sensitive services.

In a family where an isolated mother and both her children were HIV infected, all members had to attend hospital regularly for complicated medical care and treatment. The mother could not speak any English and a translator from the same community was not available. The social worker had to convey instructions about medication by drawing pictures and diagrams. This kind of situation is, clearly, unsatisfactory, and counselling virtually impossible.

In one Asian family, the father abandoned his sick wife and children because he could not accept the disgrace of his family learning of their HIV infection. Despite the fact that the abandoned mother is terminally ill, she cannot accept that there is a need to make plans for her children in the event of her death. She also fears that the school may learn of their condition and so has subjected the children to frequent school moves. Here, the common fears and paranoia associated with HIV infection are exacerbated by cultural factors. Even when a family *is* willing to receive help, close liaison and co-ordination of voluntary and statutory agencies is essential if flexible arrangements are to be made.

Because fear of disclosure is a major hindrance to care planning, it also inhibits any open discussion of the disease with the children affected. Denial is maintained – even when children are exposed to stressful events such as the death of a parent, or frequent bouts of illness. Children suffer further isolation when they are removed from school and denied normal social inter-action with their peers. Opportunities for them to express their own fears, anxieties and grief can be ignored by stressed parents who are caught up in the problems of everyday survival. The children can show their resentment, anger and confusion by increased difficult behaviour – adding to the pressures felt by parents and feeding the vicious spiral of family stress. Staff working with the children recognise that they need to spend a great deal of time exploring ways of helping children to communicate their feelings, and creating opportunities through play therapy and counselling for children to explore *their* own needs.

If present trends continue and families remain reluctant to seek help, children are more likely to be in need of foster care and respite care when they are older and sicker. Social services will have to be aware of conflicting family feelings about matching children with their ethnic backgrounds when seeking to place children with families. In general, agency childcare policies have adopted the view that transracial placements are unacceptable. Yet some minority ethnic families have already been known to refuse help on the grounds that they fear that a worker from their own community may appear to threaten their desire to withhold knowledge of their HIV status from family networks and their community.

Recruiting and training foster parents will need to be approached with great sensitivity and can only be successful if minority ethnic communities are involved in the developing of links and support networks – and if families feel that their views are treated with respect. If families are to be encouraged out of their isolation, they will need reassurances that they will not be penalised. Providing trained advocates, translators and access to information and counselling in different languages may help to breakdown barriers to communication.

Families with haemophilia

Families with haemophilia are the largest identifiable group with children who have become infected by HIV. Their infection occurred as a result of receiving contaminated Factor VIII blood products, a blood clotting agent used to prevent and to control bleeding in patients. Before rigorous blood screening programmes were introduced, it is estimated that approximately 1,000 haemophiliacs out of a population of 5,000 were infected. The number of haemophiliac male children with HIV infection under 15 years of age is approximately 190, and the same number are in their teens or early twenties.

Understanding the inherited genetic pattern of haemophilia when working with families is an important aspect of support and counselling. The disorder can be transmitted by and to both sexes but causes bleeding only in the male (except in rare circumstances). When a man with haemophilia has children, none of his sons will have haemophilia or pass on the condition, but all his daughters will be carriers – that is, they may pass on the condition to their male children, but not suffer from it themselves.[23]

Until the advent of HIV infection, families affected by haemophilia had fought hard to normalise this chronic condition, a condition which can be alleviated with medical care and treatment. They worked to be integrated into society rather than being viewed as 'disabled'. Parents have been encouraged to help their children lead more independent lives, with young haemophiliacs usually learning how to administer their own injections and take more control for monitoring their health as they reach adolescence. Close liaison has often been established with school staff so that children can usually rely on someone in school – such as a head teacher or school nurse – to support the child if there is a crisis, such as a physical accident. However, this process towards normalisation and independent living was dealt a severe psychological blow when the product responsible for liberating them, Factor VIII, became the route for transmission of a fatal disease – administered by clinical staff who paradoxically manage their on-going care and monitor their health. Most haemophilia patients and their families attend separate Haemophilia Centres or Associate Centres (there are over 100 centres) where treatment is provided. The centres were established in order to avoid treatment delays caused by travelling long distances. However, since the introduction of home therapy, it is thought that it is less necessary to live near a haemophilia centre, but that there is a case for larger haemophilia centres to be retained based on a package of comprehensive care. At these centres, patients should have direct access to a haemophilia doctor, nurse, dentist, physiotherapist, orthopaedic surgeon, rheumatologist, and social worker/counsellor. Some centres will also need to specialise in prenatal diagnosis and genetic counselling.

Many families affected by haemophilia have a strong sense of betrayal, anger and distrust because they feel that they were the victims of a medical blunder. Ambivalent feelings towards clinical staff may be reinforced by the fact that many families are currently involved in litigation with the Department of Health over compensation though they may still be largely dependent on staff with whom, traditionally, they have established close bonds or dependency relationships where several members of the same family are being treated.

Marital tensions and difficulties have been noticeably exacerbated by coping with HIV disease and the stress of living with a stigmatising condition. Problems between husbands and wives are quite common, with family tensions often involving grandparents and other children. Caring for a sick and dying child is very distressing and in some families one child may be affected but not the siblings. Siblings often need help and counselling in understanding their feelings of guilt – they may be well but feel excluded, jealous and then guilty, if all the family's attention is focused on the sick child.

Families also need sexual and genetic counselling on HIV transmission where the husband is infected, and partners need help in resolving issues concerning HIV prevention and family planning. Family needs are very complex. Traditionally mothers have played an important role in supporting children, often choosing to remain at home in order to administer to the needs of a sick child and be on call for visits to the school if a child becomes unwell. Close, over-dependent, bonds may be formed which can inhibit a child from learning how to cope with his or her condition, often leaving children shy, withdrawn and lonely. They may lack self-respect, feel resentful and may repress fears of dying – which may mirror an underlying attitude in the parents' over-protective response to his or her needs. Whereas in the past parents felt able to share information with the school about their child's condition, most parents are now afraid to let anyone know that their child has HIV infection, and will not tell family, friends or neighbours. They also find it difficult to tell their infected children or their siblings, and one of the most problematic areas for clinical staff and social workers is dealing with strong feelings of denial and anger.

These issues, related to the secrecy surrounding HIV infection, usually surface most crucially when children reach puberty – when parents *have* to confront the need to counsel children about their HIV status and offer sensitive support in helping them to cope with beginning their sexual lives. Adolescents at this stage may need independent counselling from 'neutral' advisers, in settings where young people congregate, who can offer help in thinking about safer sex and sexuality. Most professionals feel that it is wrong to delay telling children about their HIV status until they reach puberty, since many of them instinctively sense that something is seriously wrong. They need an opportunity to have their own fears and anxieties acknowledged, so that they can ask questions and begin to learn how to cope with issues related to HIV. However, some families refuse to give permission for staff to talk to children, and parental views have to be respected. When HIV infection is not handled openly within the family, tensions and crises usually erupt later. Adolescents sometimes reject the family and medical staff, refusing to attend for treatment. They are also less likely to resolve conflicting emotions and fears about their HIV condition, or to reconcile their feelings in their sexual relationships. An adolescent boy may find that he will end a relationship with a girl rather than face possible rejection if he tells her about his HIV status. Thus the difficulties of low self-esteem and social shyness may be further reinforced in haemophiliac boys with HIV. Sexual relationships can be very fraught and young couples need experienced sexual counselling and help, especially if they decide they want to have children.

Children in school obviously have a strong need to remain integrated and it is understandable that, in the light of current hysteria, parents are especially worried about breaches of confidentiality – particularly when independence and normalisation have been the preferred goals. Views from staff at haemophilia centres on how closely ties with schools should be strengthened vary. Some staff believe that it is essential if children's health is to be monitored, for there to be informed and caring members of the school staff, available to act as an emotional support if children have sudden accidents or feel unwell. However, others feel that this approach would reverse the trend towards integration and reinforce the social isolation and chronicity of children with haemophilia. The decision to inform school staff usually can only be made after full discussion and exploration of the possible outcomes with the parents and children.

Some families affected by haemophilia have experienced stigma, rejection and open hostility from local communities when HIV status has been revealed. One child was refused admission to a local school because other parents objected. The local education authority response resulted in an even more extraordinary isolation for the child – it insisted that the child be accompanied to school by a nurse who had to remain, available, in the school. Although this arrangement was later dropped after reassurance of close involvement and monitoring by the local haemophilia centre, the child is still collected and taken by separate transport to school, while his sibling travels as usual with other children. In another situation, a 14-year-old boy remained a virtual social recluse, refusing to attend school or see anyone for fear of rejection and ostracism.

Poor employment prospects and chronic illness often mean that families are already living in poverty and may be dependent on welfare benefits to supplement incomes. A higher proportion of young men of 15 years and over affected by haemophilia and HIV infection are in the poorer socio-economic bracket, compared with a similar group of men in the general population. The Social Fund has received a significant number of requests for help from haemophiliac families with HIV children. It was also found that many young men live alone and are less likely to be in stable relationships.[24]

Working with families with haemophilia is bound to remain very complex. There are legal, social, emotional, sexual and treatment problems to be resolved. Families are scattered throughout the UK, often receiving most of their primary care in small centres. Many of these are less well resourced than the major Haemophilia Centres, raising important concerns from staff, who feel that the needs of families are not always adequately met. Staff have commented that they do not always have the skills to respond to the needs for marital, family and sexual counselling.

When families and HIV infected children have to be referred to major testing centres (such as teaching hospitals) for specialist treatment and supervision of drugs such as AZT, there is a need to set up out-reach link workers – usually nurse counsellors – who can liaise with the families, local treatment centre, and local social services agencies.

Children's needs are not always prioritised and reconciling family concerns and those of the children are sometimes in conflict. There is a need to offer independent and separate counselling services for children themselves, and for more research which explores the issues from the child's viewpoint and tries to understand how *they* experience their condition.

Substitute families

Not all children with HIV infection can remain with their own families. Some will need support from substitute families when parents become ill or die, or when family support systems are not available. Support for children might include childcare daily minders, short or long term fostering, adoption, or residential care. Whatever arrangements are made for these children, all carers will need support and training in carrying out their tasks.

Experience in Lothian and other social service agencies has stressed the importance of the recruitment, screening and training of foster parents and adopters. It is essential that they are fully aware of the implications for themselves, their families, and possibly their relationships in the community if they care for a child with HIV. Carers will need an opportunity to explore whether they can cope with living with a high degree of uncertainty and stress. Carers will need training in good hygiene practices, and accurate information on HIV disease, including medical care and treatment. They need time to check out their own fears and misunderstandings, and regular sessions to up-date their knowledge. Carers will need their own support system if they are to be successful under such stress.

In Lothian it was found helpful to establish a weekly carers support group for the exchange of information and for sharing experiences. This group had links with key social work staff and easy access to medical staff, so that in times of emergency and crisis, they could quickly reach the experts. Keeping open good channels of communication was the key in enabling substitute families to cope with problems as they arose and gradually, over time, it helped them gain confidence. As time has passed, in many instances these carers have *become* the experts in caring for a child with HIV infection, and their insights on the progression of the disease have helped medical staff in understanding more about the illness. All carers will need access to bereavement counselling and support in coping with terminal illness, death and dying.

Some foster parents have established links with natural parents – offering respite care when parents become ill, or need a break. In this way it is hoped to build up continuity of care for children, if at some future date long term care is needed. A new initiative in Edinburgh in 1990 was actively involving natural parents in the selection and recruitment of foster parents. It is hoped that, with the assistance of parents, children will be placed more appropriately within their own cultural networks, maintaining a sense of their own identity and culture should they lose their own parents.

All childcare agencies involved in adoption will need to establish policy guidelines on screening for adoption. Most authorities take the view that prospective adopters will need to understand and be fully aware of HIV infection in children, but no guarantees should be made about a child's HIV status. It is not considered appropriate to screen young children for HIV infection, as testing children under two years of age is not reliable and is really only an indication of the HIV status of the mother. Parents who may be at risk from HIV infection should give their consent before any screening of children for HIV occurs. Parents' rights for confidentiality should be respected but, where known, risk factors can be shared with potential adopters, and these should be considered carefully before proceeding.

Despite early fears that there would be an increasingly heavy demand for fostering with the growth in the number of children infected with HIV, this has not occurred. The majority of children have remained at home with their own families. As the children get older and some progress to chronic illness and AIDS, or as parents become too sick to care for them, there may be an increasing need to consider alternative forms of care – such as small residential units – which may be more suitable for some children. So far, there has been no difficulty in recruiting and training sufficient foster parents, since demand has remained low. Most children who have been fostered so far have been of pre-school age – many of them being asymptomatic or in the early stages of HIV disease. However, the study revealed that there is a small but growing number of older children who will not be known to hospitals or the care system until their illness has already become advanced. Whether it will be so easy to recruit foster parents to care for older, sicker children is, as yet, untried. These children may be suffering from a range of neurological complaints; they may be more physically impaired and disabled, with loss of vision, balance and motor coordination. They could be manifesting behaviour problems connected with brain damage or be suffering from dementia. Additional difficulties will arise since, in some instances, children come from minority ethnic communities, and will need to be placed with a family from a similar cultural background.

Some authorities are already anticipating difficulty in recruiting foster parents who are prepared to take on complex care needs. At the moment one family is being supported at home by intensive daily childcare minders who look after the children whilst the parent works. However, the authority foresees that there may come a time when children will need full time residential care, where parents can visit and stay with children.

Some residential and day care units have been established in the USA, offering intensive educational and medical care support for sick children and parents. These centres are staffed by experienced teachers, playgroup workers, social workers and clinical staff. Staff work closely with parents wherever possible and share the monitoring of the child's progress, offering expert help in counselling and support for parents and foster parents. Models of 'shared care' may need to be planned in the UK, in the anticipation that *some* children will need more intensive care.

Caring for older children with HIV, who may already be in residential care, raises the same set of issues for training staff, educating them about the implications of HIV disease and offering them on-going support systems – with access to medical expertise and key social service staff responsible for HIV policies. The need to train residential care staff has already been explored elsewhere in this report, but every residential establishment must adopt clear policies in relation to caring for the emotional and physical needs of HIV children in their care. Mutual fears and anxieties about HIV *need* to be explored. One establishment coped with their concern by promoting joint training and information sessions for staff and children.[25] By creating opportunities for shared learning and openness they were able to agree on a joint set of concerns. Some issues that were identified included:

- the need to establish independent access to good medical advice and monitoring on young people's health including looking at healthy living;

- understanding their bodies;
- exploring issues of sex and sexuality;
- substance abuse;
- HIV prevention.

Information and resources for linking young people with outside specialist organisations were often unavailable. If a young person was worried about being HIV positive, both staff and residents were often unaware of local hospitals and voluntary organisations where advice and counselling could be obtained.

Much more careful planning with young people and care staff is needed in liaison with outside agencies and key social work staff in preparing a young person with HIV for independent living.

Homeless young people

There are increasing numbers of young homeless people sleeping rough in London and other cities. Even affluent West Berkshire has seen homelessness increase by 25 per cent in the last year, the largest single group being young single parents with children. Estimating the true numbers of young homeless in London is problematic and ranges from 3,000–10,000. There is no hard statistical evidence on the number of homeless who may be HIV infected, but a wealth of anecdotal evidence suggests that it may be on the increase. In addition, there is a heightened awareness of the vulnerability of the homeless to HIV infection, because of their lifestyle. Studies of the sexual behaviour of young people would support this perception. It was found that they are the least likely group to change their sexual behaviour and do not necessarily take on board messages about safer sex and safer drug use. Risk-taking is part of the youth culture and to be homeless suggests that taking risks is a way of life.

Profiles of young homeless people reveal that many have run away from care, and may have experienced several fostering and adoption breakdowns.[26] They are also more likely to have come from fragmented or disruptive family situations where physical and/or sexual abuse may have occurred. There is often a shared common distrust of adults in authority. The young homeless have experienced considerable rejection and may be low in self-esteem, have a history of disturbed behaviour, depression or even suicide attempts. Drug taking or selling sex for profit can reinforce a sense of worthlessness.

Many young people are looking for surrogate families and it is quite common to find close peer group bonds and friendships developing on the streets, where looking after each other simulates a family-type group. This group acts as a bulwark against the unfriendly outside adult world. It also acts as a powerful mechanism for socialising the new arrivals into street life mores and customs. It is not uncommon for a new arrival to be 'adopted' by an older and more streetwise adolescent who takes a familial interest in them – often acting as mentor and role model, introducing him/her to street survival techniques about obtaining drugs, prostitution, finding shelter, contacting friendly welfare agencies or engaging in petty crime. In this reconstituted family, young people are looking for the affection, closeness, warmth and support which they have missed. This informal family-type grouping and peer group support network can be a very strong socialising force in the life of street survival.

Many out-reach projects recognise that a more effective way of reaching young people in terms of health education and prevention programmes, is to target services through indirect peer group work, using the informal 'familial' network and young people themselves as 'educators' in disseminating information and advice. This approach has been pioneered in inner cities where out-reach programmes take services to the places where young people congregate. This approach implicitly recognises that potentially negative experiences can be converted to constructive responses. Consequently, reaching out to young injecting drug users and persuading them not to share dirty needles may be more effectively achieved if young people can identify with the person giving out the message. Work with young women prostitutes in Birmingham found that persuading women to practice safer sex was more effective when they used prostitutes as educators.[27]

Peer group education, however, is only one strategy. The study revealed that most agencies working with homeless young people felt totally under-resourced. There was no doubt that young people's health, psychological well-being and future prospects were permanently undermined. Work with young people often involved trying to meet complex needs when basic provision for safe and permanent accommodation remained the key problem that needed to be resolved before any other needs could be addressed. A study, by the King's Fund, of the health of homeless young families in Bayswater came to the realisation that the health care needs of young children could not be tackled until families believed that the worker was prepared to listen to their over-riding concern to be re-housed. Reaching out to young people who are ignorant, frightened and fearful of authority is an important strategy, but this has to be backed up by long-term effective policies which tackle underlying problems.

The study identified that resources should be expanded in areas such as primary health care, with 24-hour access to doctors, nurses, dentists and HIV counsellors being provided. Mobile units were identified as necessary and could include access to free needles, condoms, video and other educational material. Safe drop-in centres with facilities for childcare and offering literacy and life skills training are also needed. Special programmes for reaching under 16-year-olds involved in unsafe sex and drug misuse requires special attention. Children were reluctant to acknowledge risk behaviour because of fears of being taken into care and there was some concern expressed that very experienced counsellors were needed in sexual counselling of young people. Talking about safer sex and sexuality often raised underlying problems of young people's experience which included distressing accounts of rape, child abuse, sexual practice and activities. Work in drop-in centres had to be carefully structured so that young people could feel safe in raising issues and feel free to return subsequently to clarify problems and check out on whether to trust the worker.

Most young people needed support in attending hospital clinics, courts, and probation and welfare officers. The stigmatising behaviour of police and the prison service reinforces the view that young people who may be HIV infected will be treated inappropriately. Examples of this stigmatising behaviour are the practices of segregation and of displaying the name of a young person on remand in the prison cell on a public notice-board with the description, 'viral infection restriction'.

Services for young people tended to be fragmented, and coordination and cooperation across agency boundaries of health, social services, and voluntary organisations was unsatisfactory. The probation and prison services and housing agencies were often excluded from discussions on service developments. Care plans were often hindered by this lack of coordination, and by the different philosophies of the various agencies. Working with young drug users could be frustrating when services were not coordinated and planned following discharge from a de-toxification programme. For example, attempts to support a young woman with HIV and persuade her to seek treatment were frustrated because of the lack of adequate child minders or day care centres available for young homeless families.

The overwhelming case for a range of suitable and permanent long term accommodation to meet the needs of the young homeless has been demonstrated. This provision needs to include day care, more night shelters and crises centres, supported hostel accommodation, and more residential accommodation for vulnerable young teenagers. Additionally, drug rehabilitation programmes and childcare facilities must be an integral part of the provision for young homeless people. The impact of cutting off welfare benefits to 16–18-year-olds will have been to push some impressionable and unstable young people into increased risk behaviour.

There is a high degree of cynicism amongst agency staff about the lack of consistent policies in work with young people. The work is intensive and demanding, and has to be flexible in order to respond to the needs of young people. Only a major shift of political will and a commitment for adequate funding can hope to make any impact. In the USA, on the streets of New York it is not uncommon to see young people with HIV sleeping rough and begging. If the US model is to be successfully rejected, programmes for helping young people cannot focus only on issues related to HIV risk factors. Problems relating to HIV must be tackled within the framework of policies which really provide young people with genuine choices and options – including housing, employment and educational opportunities.

Families with special educational needs

Very little information was presented during this study about families with special needs, except indirectly through discussion with key professionals who acknowledged the difficulty of identifying whether any specific work had been undertaken on issues in relation to HIV. National organisations such as The British Institute for Mental Handicap have a working party which has been developing HIV awareness material which would be appropriate for families and children with learning difficulties.

Some children with HIV disease in the USA are already manifesting a range of developmental problems which can impair learning, affect motor coordination, and affect speech, hearing and vision. There is also experience of children developing dementia and having severe behavioural problems. So far very few cases of severe physical and mental impairments have been identified in the UK, but there is an expectation that, as medical therapies and treatments become more sophisticated and children survive longer after the onset of severe symptoms, there will be a need to develop special services to meet difficulties such as those already experienced in the USA.

Many of the agencies involved in work with families and children with special needs will have to consider how their services (and their philosophies of approach) can be adapted to take on the perspective of HIV issues in working with specialist services. A general view emerged in the study that families, special schools, and community services for people with learning difficulties were still reluctant to take on board the educational needs and HIV policy developments which would be necessary.

There is an assumption that children with learning difficulties will find it hard to understand preventive health education messages and this attitude links with parental and staff tendencies towards over-protection. Yet, in talking to teachers and workers in special education or long-stay accommodation, it is clear that sex and sexuality are major concerns that staff often find difficult to acknowledge or to handle. For instance, a day school in a busy urban area was aware that some of their young teenage girls were vulnerable to HIV infection and other sexually transmitted diseases, from casual sexual encounters that took place in the school neighbourhood. In a long stay hospital ward, adult patients were interviewed about their sexual activities and were quite open about their experiences. Denial can, however, play a powerful part in acknowledging the need for developing preventative programmes.[28]

Families will also play a part in this denial, and workers will need to be more confident in developing their own skills and knowledge about HIV before they initiate discussions with parents. Developing communication skills in working with children has already been highlighted in the study as an important gap in provision – and this is clearly even true when dealing with children with special handicaps and needs.

The implementation of statementing and strengthening of assessment of needs in the Children Act could create a useful channel for communicating information about HIV to parents and their families, and provide opportunities to explore worries and concerns. Further work in this area needs to be explored but, as a group, children with special needs are in many ways potentially extremely vulnerable to abuse and sexual exploitation and drug misuse, and there is a need to review all services involved with this care group.

5. Central government policies for children with HIV and AIDS

Central government's declared strategy on HIV and AIDS has been to prevent the spread of HIV infection by providing facilities for diagnosis, treatment, counselling and support for those affected. It has used the mechanism of ring-fenced funding to District Health Authorities and Local Authorities to develop these strategies. DHAs have to report annually on how they have spent their resources, identifying any special initiatives and developments. A review of these reports suggests that most money is still allocated to acute services – on average only 5 per cent of financial resources are spent on community services and voluntary organisations. Health education and promotion is emphasised but there is considerable overlap and duplication of functions at regional and district level. There is a lack of coherent strategies or consultation concerning the needs of children or women, except in haemophilia centres.[29]

Local Authorities have also received ring-fenced funds for the development of social care. They are expected to identify in their reports specific needs for targeted client groups, and to develop criteria for measuring outcomes – including client satisfaction and cost-effective measurements for different services.[30]

Local Education Authorities have been given ear-marked money via the Educational Support Grant mechanism to develop preventative health programmes on drug misuse through the appointment of drugs coordinators who will liaise with school staff and offer support and training to teachers – particularly in the fields of curriculum development and personal and social education. Additionally, the role of school governors in agreeing the curriculum on sex education in schools is enhanced, and every school now has to have a written policy on sex education which can be shared with parents.[31]

In reviewing these initiatives it is hard to detect any coherent strategy on, or direction in, policies for children. Health education and prevention strategies on sex, sexuality and drug misuse seem to dominate, but there is little attention given to understanding and relating to the needs, fears and concerns of the children who may be living with HIV infection or surviving in a situation where other members of the family are ill. The study revealed considerable disquiet at the lack of any formulated policy guidance on the care and treatment of children with HIV infection, especially in relation to issues affecting children in care and vulnerable young adolescents – including homeless young people and young offenders.

The need to develop coherent strategies on HIV issues for children should be led by government. Concern was expressed that, with the imminent reorganisation of health and social services, a prolonged period of upheaval and turbulence would occur. Fears were also voiced that, rather than improve standards of care for children in the health services, the reorganisation would further fragment services and reduce service provision and choice – to the disadvantage of children and families from low socio-economic backgrounds. Introducing a mixed market economy in social care could make inter-agency cooperation and collaboration *even more* complicated than at present, where coterminosity between health and local authority boundaries are already fraught with problems.

Although government policies emphasised the rhetoric of consumer involvement and choice, in reality it could be very difficult to achieve. Children with HIV infection and their families will be geographically isolated and scattered, and so can hardly be expected to present a strong consumer lobby to service providers. It is, therefore, important that government should:

- through its funding mechanism, demand more adequate reporting on how District Health and Local Authorities have targeted and assessed the needs of children and their families in relation to HIV services. Government should also require the Authorities to ensure that changes in the organisation of health services and the implementation of the Children Act 1989 include planning and integrating HIV services into mainstream provision.
- issue clear policy guidelines on the principles of good childcare practice which should be distributed to voluntary, statutory and private agencies with responsibilities for children.

Recommendations

Central Government should issue guidance relating to the needs of children concerning HIV and AIDS. It should cover aspects of:

- testing;
- legal rights of children and parents;
- consent to treatment;
- confidentiality and record keeping;
- health education on sex, sexuality, and drug misuse;
- counselling on HIV;
- bereavement counselling;
- procedures on fostering and adoption;
- care and treatment of HIV and AIDS patients;
- health and safety control;
- staff training and support;
- developing complaints procedures;
- communicating with children – including children with special needs, children in residential care, and children from minority ethnic communities;
- care planning strategies;
- guidance on legal and ethical issues;
- developing information and advisory services which address problems of communication in simple age-related language, including translation.

6. Children's needs in relation to health, education and social care

Children's needs and rights – an introduction

This chapter looks at patterns of children affected and the social provision for:

- infants and pre-school children and their families;
- primary school children and their families;
- rising teens and young people and their families.

Children's needs are explored and discussed in relation to specific groups or problems such as haemophilia, sexually exploited and abused children, drug misuse, children in care and children with special needs.

Policy trends and childcare practice are reviewed within the context of health, education and social services. However, the gulf between policy and practice is worrying and there is a need to introduce independent and rigorous screening and appraisal of standards in childcare practice.

Children should be offered child-orientated counselling services. The needs of children in residential and day care should be investigated, and specific studies should be undertaken in developing a 'participatory model' of care that identifies and incorporates the child's views and perceptions.

Educational material and information on care and treatment for children and their families should be produced in user friendly, easily understood, language. Parent-held medical records could be expanded to include agreements about treatment and social needs.

It must be acknowledged by all involved that children have the right:

- to know;
- to be consulted;
- to stay in control;
- to plan their future;
- to develop self-esteem;
- to lead a healthy normal life;
- to feel supported and not isolated;
- to have opportunities to talk to 'independent adults';
- to explore feelings about, and attitudes towards, infection status, illness, grief, loss, death and bereavement, and sex and sexuality;
- to share emotional burdens;
- to develop social skills, in preparing for leaving school and home, and exploring employment opportunities.

Diagnosing HIV infection in children

The diagnosis of HIV infection in children born to HIV positive women remains uncertain until around the age of two years when passively acquired maternal anti-bodies are usually lost. However, in some children, their immune systems may be damaged but they may not produce anti-bodies. One method for determining whether a child is infected is to identify the virus or antigen. These remain technically difficult tests and are not sensitive, so that a negative test does not mean that the child is *not* infected. More sophisticated tests are being developed but in the meantime an element of uncertainty for children and their parents will remain. There may be some children who are infected but remain undiagnosed because they remain asymptomatic. It was previously estimated that approximately one in four children born to an HIV positive mother was likely to be infected, but a more recent report of a follow-up study in ten European centres on 419 children born to women with HIV now suggests a lower transmission rate of 13 per cent. Of those babies who were infected, 83 per cent showed symptoms of infection by six months. At one year, 26 per cent had AIDS and 17 per cent had died.[32]

It is acknowledged that the number of children and women infected is likely to be an underestimate, because only those women who are at increased risk of infection are likely to be tested, so pregnant women may be over-represented. Similarly, children who acquire the virus through sexual transmission or injecting drug use rather than maternal transmission will be vulnerable, and may well be unaware of possible exposure to risk of HIV infection, and therefore unlikely to present for testing.

The progress of treatment and care of children with HIV disease and AIDS is still evolving. It is now thought that infected babies who develop AIDS rapidly could benefit most from early treatment started at two to three months, but early diagnosis is difficult.

The physical impact

When clinical disease is apparent, about 75 per cent of children present in the early stages with common non-specific signs and symptoms. These non-specific symptoms include failure to thrive or weight loss, unexplained fevers and anaemia, recurrent respiratory infections, episodes of diarrhoea, skin rashes, a runny nose, ear infections, sore throats, thrush, developmental delays and neurological impairment such as convulsions or encephalopathy. The diagnosis of AIDS in children carries a high mortality rate, with a median survival period after diagnosis of nine months. Little is known about children who remain asymptomatic but it appears increasingly likely that, with earlier and more aggressive medical intervention and treatment therapies, children will survive longer, but experience episodes of acute illness and chronic disability.[33]

Monitoring health and development

Children's health will need to be constantly monitored, and any sign of illness may trigger fears in the parents about HIV disease – and many parents will live with a high degree of anxiety about the future. With the progression of HIV disease a child may be hospitalised frequently for treatment such as intravenous immunoglobulin, antibiotic treatment for bacterial fever, and oxygen therapy. With the help of community nursing it has been possible to provide more treatment therapies at home rather than admit children to hospital. But all such treatments will require close liaison and monitoring by a paediatric team.

HIV disease can affect the central nervous system and may first show up in children as developmental delays or as signs of mental or physical impairment. Parents will also need help and advice from occupational therapists, speech therapists, teachers, educational psychologists and physiotherapists in the care and treatment of these conditions.[34]

Managing stress in children and families
The impact on the child and family living with HIV disease will affect all areas of psycho-social functioning. Children's health will need to be continuously monitored even when there are no symptoms, and any episode of illness will trigger fears and anxieties surrounding future chances of survival. Living with a life-threatening disease will cause enormous stress in parents and children, which could manifest itself in other physical illnesses in parents, emotional breakdowns, marital disharmony, and so on. Stress in children will need to be recognised and alleviated by those who have direct contact with the child in school, at home, and in health care settings. Some research in the United States has shown that it is possible to help children cope with stress and that much can be learnt from considering the behaviour of resilient children who have been subjected to hardships but have managed to function in a remarkably healthy way. Teachers, counsellors and significant others in a child's world may be able to help a child by using a variety of techniques – many of which are similar to those used in ameliorating stress in adults, but which have been adapted to be appropriate to the ages of children.[35]

Talking to children
Most of the information on HIV has been geared to promoting awareness and understanding for professional carers and parents. Children however also need opportunities to understand the nature of their illness and need the chance to have their fears, anxieties and unspoken feelings acknowledged and dealt with honestly in open discussion. Children will need considerable help in developing coping skills for living with a stigmatised condition, and will need preparation before reaching adolescence in understanding the impact of HIV disease on their physical development and how it effects their immune system. They should be taught techniques for protecting themselves from increased physical and emotional stress. Just as many haemophiliac adolescents learn to give their own injections, so young people with HIV will need to understand their medication and the importance of good diet. By encouraging a greater sense of self-control in their own health care, feelings of responsibility and maturity will be fostered and anxieties will be reduced to a manageable level. Similarly, young people will need help and guidance in relation to their own sexuality and how HIV

will affect their sexual and social relationships. This will be a difficult and testing time as young people will need to explore how they can approach issues of coping with rejection from a potential sexual partner and retain feelings of self-worth and confidence, whilst exploring personal relationships honestly and without fear of repercussions.

Information needs – involving children in decision-making

Children will need good educational and written material to help them understand their medical condition, their care and treatment – all of which must be age appropriate. They also need to understand what is involved in testing for HIV and what is meant by *consent*. Children in more vulnerable situations such as residential care, boarding schools and special schools will not always be in a position to know or ask about their care, or be aware of what they are entitled to know. In all these situations a special effort may have to be made by professional staff and carers to ensure that the rights and needs of children are central to any plans for their care in relation to HIV issues. Good practice is more likely to occur where policies and procedures exist which have been agreed and shared with staff and pupils.

One suggested model of work with children in the USA advocates an ABC approach in health education with children. This suggests that health information should be age appropriate, brief, clear, and differentiated – that is, clarifying differences between HIV infection and AIDS. The work should elicit feedback from children, give hope, and integrate information into the child's setting, inducing a willingness to hear. Finally, the educators should joke, using humour judiciously, to diffuse anxiety and discomfort.[36]

A not dissimilar approach in working with some London based school children on HIV education suggests that children should:

- be offered ways of making decisions for themselves over time;
- be offered access to information which is correct;
- be able to challenge prejudice in order to develop skills in coping and sorting out what is relevant for each individual.[37]

Working with terminally ill children

Children who are chronically ill will need opportunities to voice their views about treatment and fears about death and dying. In an oncology ward treating terminally ill children, doctors were surprised at the number of children who, when consulted, opted to cease or reduce their treatment and allow the illness to take its course. Some of these children were only eight-years-old. Experience of work with dying children has shown that children wish to be involved in discussions about their health and are often more realistic about the outcome of their illness than their parents, who will often maintain false optimism. Experienced staff working with very ill children note that this places a great strain on children since there is no opportunity for them to express their anger, aggression and fear at what is happening to them when adults insist on false cheerfulness. Helping young children to understand what is happening, and encouraging them to have more say and involvement, may be especially important in a child's ability to cope subsequently with handling fear, rejection and hostility from other children or adults.[38]

For terminally ill children it is important that they have opportunities for skilled counselling and support. Sometimes it will mean counselling children separately from their parents, who may need help in coming to terms with their own loss and grief.

Working with abused children and young people
There was considerable concern and confusion expressed in the study about the needs of children who may become HIV infected as the result of sexual abuse and/or exploitation. Concern focused on how to protect children from abusing adults who might be HIV positive, and confusion arose from ambivalent feelings towards these children who were sometimes perceived as dangerous conduits of the virus, or innocent victims of adult wickedness. All staff who work in childcare settings or in HIV services will need to be aware of policy and practice issues in relation to work with abused children. They must be aware of the implications for HIV infection, and know how to counsel and offer support.

Evidence associating HIV infection with sexual abuse or exploitation is difficult to verify. Anecdotal case histories were quite often given by staff working with vulnerable young people such as young prostitutes, drug misusers or homeless teenagers and runaways. There is considerable concern that reaching children with preventative health education measures is extremely challenging and can be almost impossible to achieve when urgent needs for drugs, shelter, food and 'bought love' will be more important to the children, than protection. Perhaps health education measures can only be successfully taken on board when long term benefits and escape routes out of a cycle of risk behaviour are planned and offered.

Concerns about testing for HIV

Issues concerning HIV and the sexual abuse of children have usually focused on the issue of testing children where HIV transmission is suspected as a result of abuse. It has been known for a child in care to be rushed off for an HIV test by anxious staff, without any considered history being taken to ascertain the known facts about the abuser. Work with abused children has demonstrated the difficulties that adults have in direct communication with children about abusing and emotionally traumatising experiences. What is *known* is that abused children will already be low in self-esteem, feel guilty, and blame themselves for the abuse – the issue of HIV infection may not be the most important problem to be resolved in working with them. Panic reactions from staff should not be tolerated and are unlikely to occur where good childcare policies and staff training have been implemented. A recent grave case of multiple sexual abuse of children, where the abuser was known to be HIV infected, led the social service department to provide a special team of HIV counsellors and social workers for the children and their families, so that support and follow-up care could be offered in a safe and confidential environment. However, where abuse has taken place, some staff working with very emotionally damaged teenage girls have counselled *against* testing, as fear, self-loathing and depression can be reinforced – and it can even precipitate a young person into suicide and self-destructive behaviour.

A test is often suggested because of fears of transmission to other adults or young people. But this should not be advocated and the problem should be dealt with by appropriate implementation of health and safety procedures and health education strategies. A test should only be suggested if it can be demonstrated that otherwise a child's health care and treatment would be impaired. Even so, testing should still only occur if the child has understood, after counselling, what is involved and gives his/her informed *consent*. Otherwise, the test itself may be seen as another form of abuse, as the knowledge of having taken the test may be entered on a child's records and subsequently have an impact on his/her chances for life insurance, jobs, mortgages, and so on.

Children in boarding schools or in care

Very little concrete evidence emerged from the study on whether there were any effective HIV policies implemented for children in private residential establishments and boarding schools. There was concern that, despite the acknowledgement that children with learning difficulties and/or special needs were vulnerable, there appeared to be scant information on how special schools were tackling HIV related issues for children, or training staff in developing appropriate educational material. Some material is being developed by voluntary organisations but there appears to be no systematic approach or generally accepted philosophy for developing policies. Issues of pastoral care, support and counselling for HIV children with special needs has not been addressed. The issue of responsibilities for children in private and boarding school accommodation and children with special needs merits a more detailed and separate study.

Communicating with children

Direct communication with children on HIV issues has been identified as one of the most difficult and challenging areas of work. Understanding the personal impact of HIV disease from the child's perspective is a crucial first stage in helping them to express their views, fears and concerns. If denial and silence are the adult's reactions in the child's presence then it has been shown by work in the USA that children are more likely to develop maladaptive defences. They deal with their problems in isolation, often experiencing self-blame, depression, denial and severe developmental disturbances.[39]

Both staff and parents often feel that they lack the skills, confidence and courage to confront HIV illness in children, and frequently express the need for more expert help and guidance in this task. Similar problems arise in work with abused children, and some of the techniques which are now being developed in this area could be transferred to work with children with HIV infection, as they will share problems associated with guilt, blame, and stigma.

The dilemmas of what to tell an infected child, at what age, how, and when are not easy to resolve. Children may need to receive information gradually over time, and in a way that leaves them with some hope and optimism. Adults face difficult and painful decisions, knowing that telling a child can make living with HIV disease more difficult. Alternatively, not telling them denies a child an opportunity to develop adaptive behaviour and explore unspoken fears and anxieties. Some children may actually find it a relief to know, as unreal fantasies and exaggerated feelings can be openly acknowledged. As children survive longer into adolescence they may need individual support and counselling from experienced staff. There should also be opportunities for 'buddying' programmes and peer group support to complement formal systems of support.

Direct communication with children should include exploring a variety of techniques including play therapy, role play, verbal and non-verbal communication, active learning through use of training materials, film, video, teaching packs and visits. There is a crucial need for good written material produced in simple user friendly language that could be used as an aid for children, parents, carers and staff. This material has to be age appropriate but should focus on practical problems and how to cope with everyday living, including taking care of themselves and advice on how to cope with difficult problems and questions.

Communicating with children must also address issues of health education and prevention, including the discussion of safer sex and safer drug use. The study revealed a clear consensus for presenting information on HIV prevention within a sex education framework, rather than focusing only on HIV issues. Responsibility for sex education has to be shared between parents, schools and the community.

Providing a continuum of care

The study identified the lack of coordinated strategies for HIV services for children and families. Children's needs will vary over time, depending on their age, their degree of disability and, various social factors. There are specific patterns of services which need to be planned and targeted for different age groups, and these are examined below – the pre-school child, the school child and young people.

The pre-school child

Developing family-centred policies

Services for pre-school children need to be highly integrated, offering a wide range of health care and pre-school provision such as playgroups, day nurseries, nursery school, and social service support for families. Some children may be showing specific signs of physical or mental impairment or developmental delays and this will call for early assessment and monitoring of a child's progress. Good pre-school services for the under fives should also enable a smoother transition to full-time schooling and allow opportunities, through good counselling, for parents and children to anticipate any problems which may arise in the school arena, because of the child's HIV status.

Services for pre-school children are best organised on a family orientated basis, an approach which recognises the importance of providing a total package of care for the family – where both parents' and children's health and welfare are interdependent. A team approach was considered essential in developing a good level of service and the study revealed a strong preference for the establishment of multidisciplinary family centres. These centres could be jointly organised and operated by staff from health, education, social services and voluntary organisations. They would undertake assessment, health care treatment and monitoring, and social care planning and support. Staff should include all disciplines, including therapists in speech, disabilities and physical impairments. Playgroup workers, child minders, volunteers and home care staff should also be integrated into inter-service provision. When children require foster care placements, there will be a need to recruit, and offer on-going support and advice to foster parents. These foster parents will be undertaking specialist work in a situation where treatment plans, care and management of babies and young children are still surrounded by uncertainties. They will also need advice, up-to-date information, and opportunities for counselling and support in dealing with high levels of stress in caring for such children. Staff and parents were attracted to this model of care because it seemed more appropriate for meeting the needs of disadvantaged communities and would be more likely to develop effective working links with hard to reach families and social networks.

Inevitably, many families will remain isolated either through ignorance, fear of discovery, or because of geographical separation. It becomes even more important that joint planning takes place at district and local authority level so that particular local patterns of need can be identified and services developed. Particular problems arise in Greater London where cross boundary movement of patients, a transient population and different agencies' policies can make the coordination and continuum of care extremely difficult.

The lack of a community based model of care which places a strong emphasis on joint planning has led to a variety of different approaches. Most of these are still at an early stage of development.

- Great Ormond Street Hospital for Sick Children has developed a model of 'shared care', where tertiary care is shared with secondary care at another hospital – usually near the family home. A community liaison nurse acts as a link with the local hospital, GPs, and social services, and, in addition, paediatricians undertake the training and education of staff in other hospitals.
- In Edinburgh, the community paediatric team is located in the acute hospital that provides support to child health clinics, home visits and liaises with social services and the voluntary sector.
- In Hammersmith and Fulham Social Services Department the HIV Unit provides a full range of services for the support and care of families with children in the community, and has developed effective liaison with health, education services and the voluntary sector.
- Haemophilia Centres are usually located as separate departments in district general hospitals. They often serve a large geographical area and patients sometimes travel considerable distances. These centres often provide a primary care service as well as offering specialist treatments such as dentistry, physiotherapy and counselling.
- In NW Thames Region a newly created consultant paediatrician is expected to act as an adviser to all the health districts, liaising with paediatric departments and community-based clinics.
- Organising community based services in a social services department can be extremely difficult. In Westminster three HIV teams service in-patients and out-patients at three major teaching hospitals. In addition, Westminster has appointed a community based social work HIV/AIDS and drugs team, a home care team, and an occupational therapy team.

The provision of out-reach work in bridging the gap in service provision may be needed for some time but it cannot, in the long run, be a satisfactory alternative for families who need more integrated and locally-based services.

The school child

Developing HIV policies in educational settings

If a good level of service provision for the under fives already exists then it should follow that the transition from pre-school to school settings should be facilitated because, in a coordinated system, communication channels with education authorities will be operating. Services developed at the pre-school stage will need to be understood and incorporated when planning services for children of school age. Yet it appears from the study that local education authorities and individual schools have been slow to adopt comprehensive HIV policies, and have failed to follow up initial DES guidance on school policies. They have neither produced specific programmes on HIV awareness nor trained staff. This has led to a state of general confusion, uncertainty and unpreparedness. Local education authorities are much more likely to develop policies without consultation with health and social service agencies, and yet there is a need for effective communication between all agencies, in order that coordinated care for children with HIV can be sustained.

The study revealed the importance of preparatory work in schools with teachers, school staff, parents and the local community in developing HIV policies for the whole school. Beginning school is likely to be a difficult time for infected children and their parents, and a crisis of confidence can be triggered off if planning prior to school entry has not occurred. For school age children important issues around integration, normalisation and confidentiality need to be addressed. These issues have always been central to the concerns of haemophiliac boys with HIV infection who, at present, account for nearly all the known cases of HIV infected children at school. This predominance of haemophilia related HIV infection will, however, gradually change as more infected children reach school age. They too will have to face a less protected environment on entering the wider world of school and on achieving increasing independence from parents.

The experience of haemophiliac families with school children infected with HIV has been chastening. Prior to HIV infection many parents encouraged doctors and nurses at haemophilia centres to develop links with the school in the belief that by sharing confidential information about the child's condition his general health and welfare could be monitored in a supportive environment. It was also felt such links could reinforce the concept of integration and normalisation, encouraging the child to experience the whole curriculum and all school activities. This philosophy was dealt a severe blow with the advent of HIV, when disclosure became associated with shame and prejudice, and the hysterical reactions of other parents. The resulting fear brought about a retraction from openness and parents are now often secretive, burdening children with the knowledge that they cannot reveal information about their infection (or that of other family members) for fear of reprisals and ostracism. These views are *not* paranoid – some children have already experienced distressing and often very public anger from local school parents when it has been inadvertently revealed that a child is infected.[40] Sometimes an education authority's response to expressions of hostility has been inappropriate. They have chosen to placate local parents by allocating special attendants to accompany a child to school or by providing additional support staff, thus reinforcing isolation and differential treatment. A more appropriate reaction would be to implement key HIV policies on confidentiality, infection control, care and support for children, staff training, and HIV health education and prevention strategies in the school.

A crucial issue for the school child and his or her parents is who, if anyone, *needs* to know about the child's HIV status. Before parents can make an informed decision on whether or not to disclose confidential information to key members of staff they should seek reassurances that the school has adopted and implemented HIV policies. If it can be determined that the school:

- has a set of clear procedures on infection control;
- has undertaken training on HIV for all staff members;
- has developed a coherent system for control of confidential information including access to school records;
- has an agreed system of offering individual support and counselling for pupils on HIV related issues;
- has consulted parents and governors in these matters;

parents may feel more confident that in the interests of the child they can consider sharing information. However, unless very strict safeguards are built into procedures, many parents will decide the risks of further psychological damage are too great – and will prefer to maintain tight control of who needs to know.

Counselling school children
Whether information about HIV status is given with safeguards or not, however, confidentiality may be breached. When this occurs, it will be even more important that there are good support and counselling systems in schools to assist children who may suffer enormous emotional traumas in coping with HIV disease and the possible reactions to it. Children who survive longer will inevitably face bouts of chronic illness, and may be subjected to an increasing range of medical therapies and intervention. There may also be increased risks of developmental delays, behavioural changes such as early dementia or increased physical disabilities which may result from damage caused by the virus to the central nervous system. Some changes may be very gradual and hard to detect, whilst other symptoms may appear quite rapidly. The impact on children could result in school refusal, self-isolation, difficulty in making friends, loss of independence, depression, educational failure, lack of confidence and poor social development. Children should have access to experienced counsellors on HIV within the school system, but it may be more appropriate if counselling and support services were also made available at other locations – including out of school hours counselling – in order to maintain confidentiality. School counselling services should liaise with educational psychologists and education welfare officers who could be involved in offering support to family members if appropriate.

Some children will find it difficult to express their fears and anxieties about their illness or dying, or discuss how they cope with everyday living – especially to friends or their family. Counselling services for school children and young people from independent agencies might be a preferred alternative. Some voluntary organisations already run telephone help lines, but often comment that there is a growing need to provide a more focused counselling service for *younger* school age children.

Counselling children in HIV related issues can also be seen as a logical extension of the school's role in health education, particularly in relation to the school curriculum. Depending on where and at what stage in the curriculum issues relating to HIV are taught teachers have often found that it is helpful if there are counselling facilities within school, particularly in secondary schools where personal anxieties or further advice may be sought.

The role of health education
The role of education authorities and individual schools in developing health education and prevention programmes is seen as crucial in helping children and young people to understand how to protect themselves from HIV infection. Teaching about HIV and AIDS in the school curriculum is a sensitive issue and is complicated further by the requirement that, under the Education Act (No. 2) 1986, school governors are responsible for deciding whether sex education should be given in schools – and in what form. Any teaching about HIV and AIDS must be affected by this requirement since it *has* to address issues related to sex and sexuality. Sex education can, however, take place in many areas of the school curriculum either as a planned topic area or through integration across subject areas.

Responsibility for personal, social, health and sex education is often split between teachers, school nurses, specialist coordinators or the newly-appointed local education authority drugs coordinators. Drugs coordinators have been appointed from the educational support grant aid to undertake specific health education work in relation to drug related problems, but they have recently had their brief extended to include a health education and preventative role in schools.

Health education is also undertaken in schools by some health education promotion units attached to the local district health authority. Policies for developing health education and preventative health care can be split between many different agencies. This task has also been carried out by leading HIV/AIDS organisations who are contracted to do the work in schools and colleges of further education where local resources are under-developed and by some local authorities who have established HIV coordinators and trainers.

This multiplicity of involvement can lead to duplication, overlapping and incoherence. Some education authorities, such as Manchester City, have established effective machinery for developing comprehensive health education strategies for the whole authority – but they tend to be the exception. Key youth organisations have also developed initiatives in out-reach work on preventative strategies but, until there is a forum where initiatives in health, education, social services and voluntary organisations can be effectively monitored and evaluated, it will be difficult to decide what the most effective role within a school should be, and where responsibility should lie.

Recent research on the effectiveness of HIV/AIDS education in schools has suggested some key elements that are important in developing successful programmes.[41] These are:

- the promotion of an active learning model where children are encouraged to explore information and issues over a period of time, clarifying knowledge and checking out anxieties;
- the key role of the teacher must be acknowledged. Ideally they should be known and trusted, and able to provide information in an open, relaxed and non-judgemental manner. The teacher should be confident in their own knowledge base and particularly comfortable in talking about sex education;
- the development of a theme approach to health education – each year taking a different topic, for example, exploring relationships – is important;
- support from the head teacher in implementing HIV education is essential;
- the importance of developing good in-service training for teachers must be realised and acted upon;
- each school should appoint a counsellor;
- good links with specialist advisers in health education appointed by the local education authority should be established and developed.

Some of the problems identified were:

- teachers lacked confidence about their own knowledge on HIV and wanted more in-service training and support for themselves;
- there was often a lack of any policy on HIV education;
- resources in schools were poor;
- there was a lack of clarity or guidance on developing HIV education in the National Curriculum;

- the development of HIV education in schools of different religious beliefs – such as Catholic or Muslim schools – has to take account of religious teachings and beliefs;
- developing HIV education in special schools was very difficult. Sometimes there were marked barriers to talking about HIV issues, and attitudes towards pupils with learning difficulties were often very protective.

Young people

There is an increase in the numbers of young people who have contracted HIV as a result of drug misuse and a growing concern that young people are less likely to change their behaviour or to practise safer sex – even when they are aware of the risks of HIV transmission. Young people are natural risk takers, and adolescence is a time when they begin to explore their own sexuality and inter-personal relationships, and start developing independent lives – away from family and school. Developing health education and prevention strategies in school is, therefore, only *one* aspect of a need for continuation and development of programmes in other areas. Particularly vulnerable young people may be those who have been hardest to reach in the school population, such as transient children from disrupted families, children in care, and those who are homeless and rootless.

The study identified the need to improve preventative health programmes in working with young drug misusers, young male and female prostitutes, and the young homeless. Work with out-reach teams and street agencies and drug programmes needed to be better integrated and planned as part of a continuum of primary and secondary health care, with improved coordination of service provision between health and social care programmes.

Young people who became HIV positive in their teens or, who survive into their teens, have special needs for counselling on care and treatment, on sexuality and safer sex, and in making realistic plans about their future. Psycho-social problems may become increasingly difficult to handle. There may also be a need to provide special respite care and small group homes to support terminally ill young people or those with early dementia. Young people in care should be given opportunities to learn about safer sex and drug use within a framework of health education.

Health policies

Developing integrated child health strategies and services

Despite a *clear* preference for a coordinated, family-centred, multi-disciplinary approach in providing HIV services, with one or two exceptions, little evidence was found by the study that this approach is being adopted. In fact, the reverse appears to be happening. Upheavals caused by NHS re-organisation predispose *more* fragmentation rather than promoting coordination in developing integrated child health strategies. Many community paediatric departments seem unclear about their future links with hospital-based clinicians and, with greater separation between purchasers and providers of health care, there is a growing concern that the natural links between services for children in the community and acute provision will be dispersed. Child health planning teams have already disappeared and community paediatricians' links with child health clinics and school health services could be further undermined by the expectation of the increased role of general practitioners in child health surveillance programmes and immunisation. Other research supports this view. Integrating child health services has proved more difficult than envisioned, particularly in inner city areas where social deprivation is directly linked to the increased need for locally-accessible child health services. One study noted that families were often presented with a confusing array of barriers because of different agencies' varying approaches and philosophies. These barriers included poor communication and coordination between agencies' and the lack of involvement of consumers in planning child health services.[42] In a recent report by National Association for Welfare of Children in Hospital (NAWCH) on setting standards for children in health care, it was stressed that each district health authority should have written policies and targets for children as a discrete client group, and should aim to integrate services for children up to school-leaving age. A planning team for children should include representatives from education, social services – and users.[43]

Continuum of care

The study revealed great confusion and lack of coherence in providing a continuum of care for children and families. The issues for care of HIV pregnant women should mean early planning and intervention so that women can discuss the future care of their children with the paediatric staff and the community services to provide on-going support and care, including services for women with a drug problem. Children with chronic ill health and handicap need long term supervision and management from social services, including education, since it has already been shown that as HIV disease progresses chidren may become impaired in speech, hearing or display signs of neurological delays.

Involving GPs

Integrated child health services would also need to consider the role of the GP in care and treatment. In a survey of GPs' attitudes to treating people with HIV, many doctors expressed a wish to be involved in shared care between hospital and home, but felt they needed more training, information and guidance on issues of confidentiality. Forty-seven per cent wanted more information on HIV and pregnancy, and paediatric HIV. It was interesting to note that the group of patients doctors felt least comfortable with were injecting drug users, a response which is of special significance for HIV parents with a drug problem[44]. An issue which may also be of increasing importance is the role of GP budget holders in prescribing. Supervising children and parents on costly drug therapies may well be considered a liability, and may result in some GPs being unwilling to treat children and/or their parents who have HIV.

Treatment issues

Treatment issues emerged as an area fraught with difficulties. One paediatrician involved in developing medical therapies described it as 'messy'. Many of the treatments for children are still in the early stages of evaluation, with uncertainties and controversy still surrounding the long-term effects of giving intravenous gamma globulin for preventing bacterial infection, or anti-viral drugs therapy such as AZT, particularly on young children. Paediatric staff felt that there was a need to develop unified guidance on the medical management of HIV infection in children, and to develop collaborative research involving other centres and clinical staff in evaluating different therapies, and in sharing expertise and information.[45]

Written information

Parents and users also wanted more explanation and written information on various treatments, and often felt confused when they perceived information was being withheld. Better communication between professionals and carers was felt to be needed. Carers wanted to be seen as equal partners in care plans, with parent-held records, and written guidance in simple lanaguage on topics such as treatment, nutrition, and care and welfare advice.

The role of the school health service

The study revealed concern and confusion about continuity of care for school chidren and the role of the school health service. Many schools reported on the reduced provision of school nurses, who in the past were seen as an important aid in supporting children with special needs and monitoring the health of children who teachers were worried about. At present the school health services are provided by district health authorities and run by community paediatricians – who form a vital link between schools and the health care system. With the introduction of child health surveillance programmes it is envisaged that most of this work could be performed by school nurses, thereby reducing the role of school doctors. There is often little or no dialogue on health issues relating to school-age children between local education authorities and health authorities, as formal machinery for cooperation and collaboration rarely exists.

The role of community paediatrics

The role of the community paediatrician is important in maintaining liaison between the hospital world of acute medicine and the more community-orientated services organised in community paediatric teams – teams who link with the child health clinics, health visitors and GPs in primary care. Community paediatricians are responsible for providing medical care and treatment, and for the monitoring of the school child. They also play an important role in issues related to assessing the special needs of children with learning difficulties or disabilities. Community paediatricians also provide medical advice and guidance to social service departments in relation to child abuse and the screening of children in fostering and adoption. The future reorganisation of the health service could seriously jeopardise the development of community paediatrics, a development which has moved it away from a medical model of care towards one of shared care in the community. The care and treatment of children with HIV infection in Edinburgh is firmly rooted in the community paediatric team approach, which favours close liaison and work with parents in the community. This preferred model for a family-centred service may not be established unless the new districts adopt policies which maintain integrated children's services.

The role of education services in developing HIV policies in school
In discussing the preferred community-orientated services response to HIV, it has been demonstrated that many schools still feel uncertain about how to handle children with HIV and will need support, training and access to good medical care and advice. Many schools revealed staff felt ill-equipped to provide advice and lacked knowledge of HIV – a situation causing some concern, considering the central role of schools. Some doctors treating children with haemophilia and HIV in haemophilia centres have offered – with the agreement of parents – to undertake this advisory role, but this *ad hoc* arrangement cannot replace the need for schools to have a whole school policy approach to all aspects of HIV which affect school children – including issues surrounding the health care of children. In assessing the health care of children with special needs, issues regarding children with HIV will need to be addressed in relation to requirements on statementing.

Guidance on the care of terminally ill children
Strong views have been expressed about the need to provide better services for the care and treatment of terminally ill children, including bereavement counselling. Staff felt that they lacked appropriate communication skills in work with dying children and needed more preparation and training. This view reflects the findings of the King's Fund, the British Paediatric Association, and the National Association of Health Authorities who have produced guidance on the care of dying children, which includes the need for regional and district health authorities to promote and publish a strategy for the care of children with life-threatening conditions. The findings suggest that all districts should provide domiciliary paediatric nurses who will liaise with the hospital and the home, offering shared care to parents and children. It also suggests that each district should have a named officer responsible for services.[46]

Summary

Current health policies for HIV children and parents are fragmented and underdeveloped, with the responsibility of care divided between too many different acute specialities and community services.

All District Health Authorities should urgently review policies and services for children with HIV – but within a framework of *integrated* child health services.

Services for women with HIV must recognise the preference of parents for locally-based family-centred clinics which can provide a range of care, treatment and supervision for infected children and parents, and which can also offer rehabilitation services for drug using families in parallel with counselling and support services.

Education policies

The study revealed considerable disquiet at the apparent lack of detailed planning and promotion of HIV policies in schools, despite excellent work pioneered in some areas. Some local authorities have taken a proactive stand and have seen their role primarily to stimulate and encourage the development of health education and health prevention strategies both within schools and out of school, in formal and informal settings where young people congregate. Some authorities have established joint coordinating committees, usually forming liaisons with health education units of health districts, youth organisations and voluntary groups. It was less common to find evidence of joint strategic work with education and social service departments or with all three services of health, education and social services.

The Department of Education and Science (DES) issued early guidance to education authorities in 1986 in a document called, *Children at School and Problems Related to AIDS*. This guidance established the parameters of issues relating to HIV transmission, safe hygiene practices, counselling and confidentiality, care of children with HIV in the school (including the management of handicapped children), children's games and social practices, and health education. In addition, the Health Education Authority (HEA) and DES provided teaching packs and a video for use in schools. This guidance makes it clear that children with HIV infection should be integrated into all school activities, and that HIV status is *not* to be considered as grounds for excluding any child from access to school.

Despite the early publication of this guidance, however, it still appears that education authorities have not been successful in following it up with more detailed implementation of HIV policies in schools. Neither have they promoted staff training nor clarified roles and functions in schools concerning HIV policies. Reports from the survey suggest that school staff did not feel confident in their knowledge and understanding of HIV/AIDS, or even know what groups of staff *had* received any relevant in-service training. Support staff – such as administrators, domestics, play ground assistants, school porters, and meals supervisors – all play key roles in relating to children but may not have had opportunities to discuss HIV policies.

Issues relating to confidentiality have often not been properly addressed and remain controversial. Guidance suggests that the rights of children and parents for privacy should be respected and that the number of people, including teachers, who are informed of HIV status should be restricted to those who *need* to know in order to ensure the proper care of the child in the event of school injuries or accidents. Many teachers, on the other hand, expressed different views and felt that they *should* be informed about a child's HIV status in order to protect both other children and the infected child. Some teachers also worried about the levels of their skill and knowledge in supporting and counselling children with the virus, and their parents, and felt that they would need more skilled support and expertise from medical and social work staff in carrying out this task.

Issues of confidentiality also touched on whether school systems of record keeping were adequate, and whether the procedures on confidential information were agreed by schools or the education authority. The relationship of a school with the community it serves was also raised as a key issue in developing HIV policies. Despite an agreement on confidentiality, problems may arise such as when some parents in small or rural communities have learnt of a child's HIV status and have threatened to boycott schools if the child was allowed to attend. In order to avoid such a confrontation, there was a need for the school, the education authority and the social work department to provide community HIV awareness sessions for parents, and to educate parents, teachers and governors about HIV transmission. This approach turned a potentially hostile situation into one that welcomed the child and also provided special support staff to the school. In contrast to this approach, a different local education authority in response to a similar situation insisted that a special school nurse attend daily and was expected to be present in the classroom with the child involved.

The importance of schools formulating clear policies on infection control and confidentiality procedures, providing staff training, and ensuring support for children cannot be overstated. In addition, it is essential that schools involve local parents and school governors in HIV awareness training sessions and discussions, and explain school policies on HIV. Opportunities should be created for school policies on HIV to be aired and a consensus reached on how to address *all* of these issues. In this way, crisis decision-making is more likely to be avoided and future difficulties anticipated.

Health education in schools is seen as an important conduit for developing awareness in children about HIV transmission and preventation, and it can be taught at different stages and in many subject areas of the curriculum. However, a favoured approach in schools is to include teaching about HIV and AIDS within the broader context of the personal and social education curriculum, and as an integral part of sex education. Under the Education Act (No. 2) 1986 it is now the duty of the school governors to decide whether or not sex education should form part of the secular curriculum of their school. If it is agreed that sex education should be a part of the school curriculum, governors have a duty to agree the content of the curriculum and to produce a written policy for the school on its sex education programme. This policy should be published and made available to parents. There are many critics of this approach, and some believe that it is difficult to develop appropriate health education measures if teaching about sex and sexuality is not seen as an important framework for discussing inter-personal relationships. Alternatively, others feel that by involving school governors in the discussion, it is more likely that open and constructive debate on important and related health prevention strategies will be fostered.

In evaluating an in-service programme for teachers on learning about HIV, it was revealed that teachers themselves felt de-skilled, lacking in confidence and unsure of their communication skills in talking about sex education and HIV prevention. Most teachers wanted more in-depth training, support and help in developing sex education materials. Teachers agreed that the most important strategy in class-room teaching was to focus on student-centred learning, an approach which was considered more appropriate than didactic, pedagogic methods.[47]

Other important areas of HIV policy in schools needed clarification and they included dealing with the confusion over roles and responsibilities in relation to health education. Traditionally in some schools it had been considered part of the school nurse's role. In many schools, however, the main responsibility now lies with the named teacher in charge of the personal and social education curriculum. In some authorities drug coordinators have been established to liaise with schools in developing awareness about drug misuse and educating children about drug use prevention. Some co-ordinators are now expected to extend their responsibility to cover all issues of HIV prevention. There is a great variation in the level and range of LEA provision in relation to youth and community education services. Some LEAs have developed comprehensive HIV policies and strategies for young people out of school, but in general this is a neglected area. There is a need for LEAs to develop HIV policies for all their departments but especially for young people in the community, and more effective liaison with voluntary and statutory organisations should be established. A similar confusion arises over offering support and counselling for children with HIV or those who have personal worries about related issues. Not all schools yet have a named person, but it is strongly recommended that all schools identify a key person who will undertake counselling duties.

It is still unclear whether educational psychologists, education welfare officers and school health support services such as speech therapists, school doctors and dentists, have clarified their roles and functions in relation to the needs of the school child – HIV infected or not. In particular, education authorities have been slow to implement guidance and training for staff working in special education. Unless education authorities promote the regular review of school policies on HIV and provide adequate resources for in-service training and support services, an important opportunity to provide on-going preventative health measures, care and support for children with HIV will be lost. The role of the school health service in relation to medical care and supervision of children with HIV is confusing, and the situation was discussed more fully in the section on *The school child* on page 62.

Summary

All education authorities should review the effectiveness of the HIV policies and procedures operating in their establishments.

Education authorities and District Health Authorities should consider developing joint strategies on health education and preventative programmes, as there is still considerable overlap, duplication and confusion about different roles and responsibilities.

Education authorities should review with district health authorities the role of the school health service as part of the development of coherent child health services for the care and treatment of children with HIV.

Particular attention should be paid to the following areas of HIV policies in schools:

- improved in-service training for teachers should be developed, especially in relation to communication skills in talking about sex and sexuality;
- all school staff should be given the training they need in HIV awareness;
- parents, governors and the local school communities should be involved in developing community education programmes on HIV;
- confidentiality procedures should be agreed, including guidelines on the recording of information;
- schools should appoint a named person to act as counsellor for children with HIV worries;
- education authorities should explore providing a borough-wide counselling and support service for all children;
- the needs of children in special schools should be considered a priority, and the urgent development of appropriate educational programmes or materials acknowledged as essential.

Social service policies

Social service organisations have a pivotal role in providing and co-ordinating care in the community for children and families with HIV infection. In carrying out this task they liaise with the voluntary sector and other statutory bodies – particularly health, education, housing, and social security departments. They undertake a complex range of duties in association with their statutory responsibility for the care and protection of children, statutory duties which are enshrined and expanded in the Children Act of 1989. This legislation addresses issues which have emerged as crucial in developing HIV policies for children and young people. In particular the Act emphasises shared responsibility and partnership between social services departments, and parents, carers or guardians, and also displays an enhanced regard for the rights and wishes of the *child* in an assessment of needs and the making of care plans.

The most important issue in relation to the role of social services was identified in the study as the need to clarify areas of good childcare practice when developing HIV policies and services for children and young people. Social services provide a range of services for children and their families including day care services such as day nursery, child minding, day centres, and home care; fostering and adoption; social work support in hospital and community settings; and a range of residential child care provision. Good childcare policies should espouse the philosophy of normalisation, equal access and non-discriminatory provision. However, in reviewing the development of HIV childcare policies during this study, it was difficult to identify any consistency of approach. The study revealed widely differing standards and it was only in areas of proven need – such as Scotland and other centres – that strategic reviews of childcare policies had led to the development of a coherent set of HIV policies for children.[48] This lack of consistency inevitably leads to bad childcare practices. There were numerous examples presented during the research which illustrated the problems which arise when inappropriate staff responses have triggered a distressing sequence of events. Children in residential care have been tested without their knowledge or consent, sometimes on flimsy heresay evidence, before ascertaining risk factors or discussing implications of testing with the young person. Some babies have been tested for the virus without obtaining parental consent or the consent of the Department. There have been appalling breaches of confidentiality, for example one child continued to test negative over several years but the original record of testing remained on the file – thus sustaining an association of stigma. In another case, an HIV positive parent who's child was in a day nursery was confronted by an angry day nursery worker who had learnt of her HIV status from reading her records. A foster parent, involved in a different case, learnt that the parents of the child she was fostering were HIV positive, and, though the child's status was unknown, she insisted on the child being removed.

Good childcare practices are more likely to be developed where effective policies and procedures lay down clear lines of accountability in decision-making and where the wishes and views of children, parents and carers form an integral part of planning services. Because information on care and treatment of children with HIV is changing continually, all HIV policies will also need to be reviewed and up-dated regularly in consultation and liaison with the developing policies in health, education and the voluntary sector.

The crucial issues which must be addressed in formulating HIV policies have been referred to constantly in other chapters and sections of this book and so are taken as read. Many social service departments have implemented HIV policies broadly based upon these issues, however they should also include specific references to *how* these policies will be interpreted in work with children and their families. A good model of such policies and their interpretation has been developed by Hammersmith and Fulham Social Services Department HIV Unit, and is being up-dated to include relevant amendments on work with drug using parents and to take account of the requirements of the Children Act.[49]

Because so many aspects of care are inter-related and require joint strategies and multidisciplinary team work, there is bound to be some overlap and duplication of service provision. This is particularly true in developing services for drug misusing families and young people, health education and prevention strategies, and counselling services. If joint policies and strategies are established in cooperation with health, education and the voluntary sector, it will be easier to identify the key people who may be the most appropriate in providing a particular service. An added advantage to be gained from this approach is that it should also facilitate the sharing of expertise and knowledge.

The following sections outline specific areas which should be covered when developing HIV policies.

Confidentiality

Procedures for dealing with issues of confidentiality should establish the legal rights and professional medical issues involved, including guidance on what constitutes consent to share information. Procedures should define the circumstances under which information can be shared – and with whom. Central to all matters of confidentiality are the rights of the individual affected to control who knows and for the decision to *remain* with them. The consent of the parents or guardians must be obtained before HIV status is divulged, unless to withhold consent is deemed to be harmful to the child's interests. Where an infected child is old enough to understand, their consent should also be sought. Confidentiality procedures on *all* record keeping should be established and staff administrators trained to handle sensitive matters.

Testing

Procedures laid down for testing should cover all aspects, including counselling for parents and children at both the pre- and post-test stages. Children should not be tested without their informed consent unless there are overriding reasons for doing so – such as protecting their health or that of others. Clear accountability procedures need to be established which set out management decision-making structures and locate how decisions are arrived at and who is responsible for them.

Counselling

Counselling on HIV issues should be available as a key area of service. Children will need on-going support and help, especially as they reach adolescence and at times of crisis. Counselling services for children could also include a telephone helpline. The service should be well publicised and should be seen as an independent, arms-length service. Families with HIV and foster parents caring for children with HIV will also need counselling support from time to time especially at times of bereavement or loss, or when resolving stress within the family caused by living with a stigmatised condition.

The care plan

In drawing up any care plan for an individual child or young person with HIV Hammersmith and Fulham SSD suggest the following principles should be considered:

- what are the physical, emotional and development needs of the child?
- what are the expected levels of interaction with other children?

- what are the benefits and disadvantages to both the HIV positive child and others of any particular placement or service?

Managing medical and social care

This calls for a thorough understanding of the progress of HIV infection in babies, children and young people. Staff must be familiar with medical therapies, clinical signs and up-to-date treatment issues. Parents, foster parents and care staff in all settings will need training in recognizing the care needs of children and support in providing practical help in maintaining both the child's well-being and that of the family including written information. This will include assessment of needs, the provision of additional money for special diets, laundry facilities, home care support, respite care, transport, holidays, or additional payments for special needs. Aspects of social care should include the provision of services such as developing support groups for foster parents and adopters, children and/or their parents. Liaising with voluntary bodies particularly those caring for young people or drug misusing families in community based projects and street agencies is another important aspect of statutory social care provision.

Staff training

This is an essential cornerstone of HIV policies for children. Staff will need opportunities for in-service training and regular reviews of training needs. In particular, staff providing direct care and support for children with HIV must be familiar with departmental HIV policies, and should receive training on aspects of HIV transmission – including practical help in communicating with children on issues related to sex education and drug misuse. Training strategies should include peer group review, staff support and supervision, evaluation and monitoring. Guidance on the training needs for all social services staff has been published by CCETSW (*Living and working with HIV*).

Support for carers

Foster parents, carers and volunteers will need support and, possibly, specialist training in undertaking demanding work in caring for children. Foster parents may need to be specially recruited to care for children with special needs who become chronically sick and disabled or who may have severe behavioural problems. Regular support and counselling will be necessary and provision must be made for access to emergency services and expert help in times of crisis. Respite care will also need to be organised to relieve relatives and other family members who may be caring for several sick members in one family.

Health and safety

Everyone involved in the care of children such as:

- childcare staff;
- foster parents;
- adopters;
- playgroup workers;
- nursery staff;
- volunteers;
- childcare minders;

should receive training on health and safety procedures that are consistent with standards required for preventing HIV transmission. This should include written information and access to health and safety advisers.

Special needs

Some children may become chronically ill or have special problems which require intensive residential care, or day care support. They may become physically impaired, lose coordination, or be unable to walk. They may be visually impaired or develop educational or behavioural problems due to neurological damage. Providing specialist services will require staff skilled in nursing, occupational therapy and educational techniques. Policies should be developed that can make provision for special care for a select group of children who may not be able to remain in their own homes.

Drug policies

Policies in local authorities and health and social services departments need to be coordinated in working with drug related families and children. Working with drug-using families is an increasing part of HIV work – an acknowledged growth area. There is a need to be clear about departmental strategies and policies on drug-related problems and to review these in the light of appropriate local service provision and support for families.

Communicating with children

Direct communication with the clients is a neglected area of work in all aspects of services for children. Policies for children should recognise their individual rights to be consulted and to have their views respected. Children should be *involved* in decisions about their care and treatment and should be *informed* about their rights in regard to consent to treatment, testing and confidentiality. Information should be provided for all children in care and should be presented in simple language that they can understand. It should also inform them of how to obtain independent advice and information, and should include a named individual to whom they can go for counselling or advice.

Acknowledging the need of children for independent counselling, support and advice if they become infected is crucial, and provision of this kind should be built into the policies for providing services to children. Staff will need to develop skills in communication by exploring a variety of teaching techniques and methods and the use of various materials.

Children in residential care

The care and management of children in residential care and children with special needs was considered to be the most under-developed aspect of HIV childcare policies. This is an area of great neglect. All children in residential care should be included in discussions about HIV departmental policies and should be informed of their rights. Too many care establishments react with ill-informed and prejudicial attitudes. This is an area of work which should receive priority in developing effective training strategies for staff, with opportunities for regular in-service training and up-dating to maintain training levels.

Issues in relation to HIV prevention strategies and sex education are surrounded with feelings of moral panic and incoherence, with staff often having few skills in health education or much experience of relevant teaching techniques. High staff turnover means that young people may have few stable adult figures who can effectively help them in exploring interpersonal relationships.

HIV policies in relation to residential childcare work should be reviewed, and staff should be given clear guidance on these policies. Expert support and staff supervision in exploring ways of working with children and young people should also be provided.

Monitoring services

All services for children with HIV and their carers should be regularly reviewed and monitored. This monitoring should include representations from both user groups and the voluntary sector.

Complaints procedures

An important and necessary adjunct of good monitoring is the provision of a complaints procedure where problems, and complaints about services and practice, can be effectively resolved. Children in particular may need help in processing complaints as they will often feel very vulnerable and will need independent advice. Appointing independent advocates for children should be a considered option, though this may well be more appropriately undertaken by a voluntary childcare organisation.

Summary

Social services departments should initiate and develop joint strategic planning with health, education and the voluntary sector in providing a range of HIV services for children and their families. Social service departments should review their policies on HIV and ensure that specific guidance on all aspects of childcare policy and practice is included. This guidance should take into account the Children Act 1989.

All staff working with children should be required to undertake specific training on communicating with children, and should have access to expert childcare professionals.

7. The role of voluntary organisations

Voluntary organisations have played a major part in developing and pioneering the emergence of a range of new services for people who are HIV positive. Based on some of the early American experiences, these groups can be characterised by their embrace of a more consumer-orientated approach – one which seeks to empower previously stigmatised and disenfranchised groups such as gay people and drug users. By encouraging user involvement in the planning and running of services, they have forged important links with powerful advocates in health and social services who have begun to recognise the benefits that accrue to clients' general well-being when they are centrally involved in decisions about their health and welfare.

Whether the consumer voice will be sustained as HIV organisations broaden the basis of their work to incorporate the needs of women, children and families is as yet untested. Some voluntary women's organisations have argued that women are less likely to join in active campaigns or lobby for improved HIV services because they fear reprisals, victimisation and social isolation for themselves and their children. They may be reluctant to join self-help groups, may lack self-esteem, and often may be less mobile because of family responsibilities. In addition, they may be ill themselves and have few local support systems. Voluntary organisations will need to be aware of these differing needs and to respond flexibly – developing local networks of services which are family-centred, non-stigmatising and accessible. Some organisations have already pioneered services for young women and children in drug rehabilitation – services which seek to normalise their lives in the local community by supporting them over a sustained period of time, thus helping them to develop independent life skills and self-confidence. This work is, however, labour intensive and calls for high levels of both staff support and resources.

A noticeable feature of much voluntary work at the 'coal face', whether it be with the young and homeless, drug misusers or families with HIV and haemophilia, is the time lag between identifying needs and persuading funding bodies to provide adequate financial support. Local Authorities and District Health Authorities are often major sources of funding for the voluntary sector, yet many still do not have any clear criteria or policies for liaising and working with voluntary organisations. There is clearly a need for national voluntary bodies to support and campaign effectively for a more coherent funding strategy, one which recognises and adequately funds new initiatives.

Although services for adults with HIV are now well established and voluntary organisations such as The Terrence Higgins Trust have articulated and campaigned most effectively on behalf of adults, there is still no childcare organisation fulfilling a similar role at national level for *children* with HIV, although Positively Women are in touch with many women and chidren and their needs.

Some voluntary organisations, however, have led the way in pioneering new services for children and families with HIV such as The Aberlour Child Care Trust and the Mildmay Mission. Work has also been undertaken by Save the Children Fund (SCF) and the National Council of Voluntary childcare Organisations (now called childcare) on developing HIV policies and strategies for staff and children. Barnardo's has reviewed all its services and is intending to establish specific services for bereaved children and families including placement of children in foster homes. But in general there appears to be no coherent approach or focus from the voluntary sector. The survey revealed that many national childcare organisations had not yet begun to address HIV related issues specifically in respect of children in any systematic or sustained way. There was also a marked difference in organisations primarily working in services for the under fives and their families and those working with older children in care or with special needs or disabilities.

Organisations working for the under fives were more likely to have developed policy guidelines covering aspects of health and safety, confidentiality, testing, fostering and adoption, training, and childcare practice. Many of them have published information and leaflets for staff, carers and user groups. They were also more likely to have developed training strategies and initiated project work. In contrast, organisations concerned with older children and children in residential care or with special needs or disabilities seemed less prepared. Some national organisations are now beginning to develop policies and initiate training, but typically there did not appear to be any sense of urgency until confronted with a crisis. This usually arose following an incident where a child or young person in care was 'perceived' to be 'at risk' from HIV infection, and often resulted in staff reacting inappropriately and sometimes submitting children to HIV testing procedures – with little understanding or awareness of the outcome of such a test on the child's well-being.

Concepts of 'care' or 'control' are often not resolved when considering the needs of children in relation to HIV. Work to understand the spectrum of needs of children with HIV has hardly begun, with much of the current knowledge having been gleaned from work with young children born to HIV infected mothers. There are, however, considerable numbers of school children and young people already living and coping with the virus in the community. More detailed knowledge of how they cope, and what their needs are, would help to shift the balance from the 'control' aspect of work with children with HIV to that of caring. Some of this work is undertaken by the Haemophilia Society but their resources are very limited and the needs of children have to compete with other demands on the Society's time. Similarly, voluntary organisations working with young people are more likely to have limited resources of time and staff and often feel overwhelmed by the complexity of expressed needs.

Voluntary childcare organisations are responsible for the welfare of well over 100,000 children and can often reach out and offer services more flexibly to meet local community needs. They should be playing a more major role in educating their own organisations, developing social policies for children with HIV, and stimulating research and discussion about current policies and future needs. In particular, they should pioneer research into improving skills and techniques in direct communication with children. This is already a contentious issue in work with abused children and many of the dilemmas faced in working with children with HIV are similar. Indeed, some young people will acquire HIV infection as the result of sexual exploitation or abuse by adults. This makes it doubly difficult to develop relationships of trust with other adults, and has major implications for developing social and personal health education programmes which enhance self-esteem and self-worth.

Recommendations

- Establish a Standing Committee of Childcare Organisations to act as a forum for stimulating discussion, information exchange and research, and for monitoring the development of all aspects of HIV policy in relation to children and their families.
- Specific research should be undertaken which evaluates:
  – what makes for effective communication with children;
  – how does it take place;
  – how well services handle this process.
- Publish guidelines on HIV Childcare Policies to all childcare organisations, establishing principles of good childcare practice. These guideline policies should cover aspects of health and hygiene practice, facts about HIV, confidentiality, testing, fostering and adoption procedures, staff training, non-discriminatory practices, and codes of practice, including disciplinary procedures.
- Establish more accessible material and information for the users of services, such as families, carers, foster parents and adopters, and volunteers.
- Develop criteria for the funding of the voluntary sector by the statutory bodies through liaison. Establish a clearing house for quick access to emergency funding for smaller pioneering agencies, who are often working without resources or support. Develop criteria and procedures for the resourcing of special needs – such as holidays, respite care, housing, diet and so on.
- Organisations working for children with special needs and disabilities should be encouraged to develop special educational programmes and material on HIV issues which are appropriate to the needs of staff, carers and children.

8. Training

Training on HIV/AIDS was seen as an important priority in preparing staff to work with confidence and competence in HIV services, but training needs sometimes appeared to be at variance with agency policies and practice on HIV. Many agencies saw their responsibilities for preparing staff as being fulfilled if they issued them with written policies and guidelines. Staff commented that training sessions were often limited to HIV awareness days and did not allow sufficient opportunities to update knowledge and develop further skills to a greater depth. Resources and training budgets were also often very limited, and smaller voluntary organisations complained that they could not afford to send staff on HIV training courses.

Whilst many agencies felt that they had acquired some basic information and facts about HIV, very few felt confident in dealing specifically with areas of need for babies and children with HIV. Others felt it was important to widen their understanding of working with families where several members might be ill. Knowledge about chronic illness in children and issues concerning working with young dying children and bereavement counselling were, however, considered important. Many staff expressed the need to develop skills in working with drug misuse – misusers themselves and their families. Agencies felt that staff needed continuing opportunities to update knowledge in order to take into account the changing needs of clients and staff turnover.

Training approaches varied both within individual agencies and between different types of agencies. For example, social services departments already involved in developing services for people with HIV in areas of high need were more likely to have developed training programmes for staff, although not all of them would have necessarily trained foster parents or childcare staff. Departments such as Lothian in Scotland, and Hammersmith and Fulham have developed training strategies for staff which coordinate agency policies on HIV positive children, young people and families. Lothian has also pioneered intensive training for foster parents, carers, support workers, and potential adopters.

Voluntary organisations catering mainly for young children and the under fives were also found to be more likely to have developed training strategies and policies for staff than organisations working with older children. Training for staff working with children in care or in special residential schools, however, was considered inadequate and, in many instances, had not been provided at all. Many staff, however, were aware of deficiencies and acknowledged their lack of knowledge about HIV procedures, particularly on testing young people, drug misuse and safer sex counselling. Implementation of the new Children Act of 1989 has emphasised the importance of improving the training of *all* childcare staff, particularly in relation to working with sexually abused and exploited children. Knowledge about HIV issues in relation to children should be seen as an *integral* part of the curriculum in addressing childcare needs.

Training strategies for staff working in the education services appeared to be less systematic, and it was often difficult to locate any line management responsibility for training staff. Concern was expressed at the lack of in-service training for teachers, school nurses, school doctors, dentists and ancillary staff. Some local education authorities (LEAs) had developed a multidisciplinary approach to training school staff in cooperation with local health promotion units, but others appeared to have adapted a *laisser-faire* approach. Teachers expressed concern about the lack of general HIV policies in schools – many had received little information apart from an early circular from the DES. They also expressed concerns about issues relating to confidentiality and to their role in counselling the parents of children with HIV. Targeting training in schools often appeared to be negotiated on an *ad hoc* basis, rather than as a consistent policy initiative from the Education Authority covering all schools in a locality. There were examples of work with children with special needs, such as deaf children, but it was not always clear whether the focus of the work was on training staff, or on educating children about HIV issues.

Surprisingly, many health care staff also commented on the general lack of training opportunities on HIV and, in particular, were concerned that they were not sufficiently well-informed about current models of treatment and intervention for children with HIV. This problem was acute in districts located some distance from the main HIV treatment centres, where only a few children had been identified as HIV positive. Paediatric staff also expressed concern about their current knowledge and expertise, and felt particularly that they would need additional training on bereavement counselling and working with dying children.

Training children, young people and parents

Two groups which training strategies usually ignore are those of the children themselves and their parents. Training parents on how to care for their children and enhance their own skills is not much in evidence, with the exception of training for foster parents, and yet some of the smaller voluntary organisations working with parents and young children have emphasised the *importance* of involving parents in training. The effects of parental training are felt to be self-evident since, as they become better informed and skilled in caring, trained parents can, through peer-group education, reach out and 'train' other parents and carers.

As with parents, very little training is offered directly to children and young people – particularly those living in residential care or schools, and children with special needs or disabilities. Experience in residential units for adolescents, however, has shown the vital importance of educating young people about HIV so that they can both protect themselves, and also understand the needs of a young person with the virus. A child or young person with HIV may suffer rejection and stigmatisation from others unless young people in care have an opportunity to explore HIV issues for themselves. Developing training programmes for young people in care will require detailed knowledge and assessment of the needs of particular groups of children, so that material can be adapted to meet these needs – producing it in a form that is relevant and appropriate. It will also require adult trainers to work in close cooperation with the staff of residential establishments and schools to ensure that training opportunities are supported – and are developed – within the context of good childcare practice.

Training policies rarely mentioned the need to train volunteers, although many of the HIV voluntary agencies have pioneered the development of training programmes for volunteers. As service needs expand, the need for volunteer training will increase.

Recommendations

- Agencies should develop coherent training strategiees on HIV/ AIDS which address the needs of staff in preparing them to work in HIV services. Training strategies should be an integral part of HIV policies and service developments.
- Specific training budgets and resources should be allocated for HIV training in agencies. Training should be evaluated and monitored, and staff training needs regularly assessed and updated.
- In-service training is an important part of service developments and should be offered to all new staff.
- Agencies should identify a key person who is responsible for training, particularly in residential establishments.
- More trainers from Black and minority ethnic communities are needed and agencies should ensure that the training needs of Black and minority ethnic staff are addressed.
- Specialist training and modular training on work with children and families with HIV is needed.
- Training programmes should be developed for carers, foster parents, parents, young people, and volunteers.

Specific areas to be covered in training
- Facts about HIV transmission in children and young people, including the process of disease, symptoms, care and treatment.
- Information on agency policies and procedures on HIV, which should include testing, confidentiality, non-discriminatory policies and equal opportunities.
- Specific policies on childcare practice, covering aspects of children in care, fostering and adoption procedures, and the role of carers.
- Health and safety procedures, including good working practices in infection control.
- Addressing attitudes and feelings about HIV/AIDS which covers issues related to stigma, prejudice, guilt, death, bereavement,

racism, cultural and religious diversity, sex and sexuality, and drug misuse.

- Skills in communicating with children and young people, including direct work with sick and dying children.
- Understanding issues related to drug policies, including harm minimisation and alternative treatment approaches in drug misuse.
- Addressing the issues of sex education and sex and sexuality, within the context of health education programmes.

9. Professional issues

Living with uncertainty is a key feature of HIV work which covers all aspects from uncertainty about medical care and drug treatments, predictions about the scale of the epidemic, or forecasting the long-term social impact of HIV on individuals and communities.

Consideration of these issues has begun to challenge areas of professional practice, values and assumptions which previously may have been taken for granted. This is evident in discussions relating to confidential information, consent to HIV testing and treatment, and sharing professional knowledge with consumers. As a consequence there is being seen a growing sensitivity by some professionals in understanding and acknowledging the limitations of their role, and in conceding the importance of recognising the rights and needs of consumers – and their contribution in power sharing.

The following areas of concern were mentioned most frequently.

Organisational issues

Lack of HIV strategies and policies

There was considerable criticism of the organisational response to HIV in all settings. There were 'beacons' of good practice but these only heightened awareness of the gulf which exists between informed agencies and the rest. Staff complained that they felt ignorant, vulnerable and unsupported, as they were often operating services, without any policies or guidance from their organisations. Many had a limited awareness of government policy directives on important areas such as confidentiality, HIV testing, or health and safety procedures. Remarkably, even where procedures existed, they varied even within the *same* agency – it was common to find that different departments in a hospital or social service agency, for example, were implementing inconsistent policies on health and safety procedures or confidentiality.

Conflicting philosophies

Professional goals and tensions, inconsistencies, and different philosophical approaches were often most marked in hospital settings. This was dramatically illustrated in one district where clinical medical staff wished to test *all* women attending ante-natal clinics for HIV infection, without informing the patients. This was bitterly opposed and fought by the midwives who upheld their professional doctrine of opposing testing without consent, as this was considered an 'assault' on the patient, and midwives could be subjected to disciplinary action if a patient complained. Professional guidance has been issued by many professional associations, but this is easily undermined in the workplace if organisations fail to clarify the philosophies and principles which guide their services. These principles and philosophies held by organisations should be scrutinised and open to challenge by consumers if they wish to exercise this right. Some authorities, such as Hammersmith and Fulham Social Services Department have published a manual on policy and practice guidelines which describes exactly what procedure should govern services for HIV positive children and young people who are diagnosed as being HIV positive. It covers aspects of confidentiality, testing, care and management, issues for carers, staff recruitment, and training on health and safety.

Uncoordinated services

There were complaints about managerial remoteness and poor communication between professional groups and their hierarchies. Some felt isolated and lacked access to appropriate information, resources or training. Experienced staff stressed the importance of developing good liaison machinery between all care givers so that advice and treatment for women and their children was consistent. This was especially true for women with HIV during and after birth, who needed support and advice from a team of staff including, doctors, nurses, immunologists, counsellors, community paediatricians, health visitors and social workers. Coordinating care between different agencies was considered crucial in developing integrated child health services, but there was a general pessimism on how this was to be achieved since the demise of most of the children's health care planning forums in the NHS. Many thought that the fragmentation of services would worsen with the introduction of the new NHS and Community Care Act in 1990.

Professional isolation in schools

Teachers seemed particularly isolated and were mainly unaware of their local education authorities' policies – or even if they *had* any on HIV issues in relation to school children, staff training or school policies. There were examples of interesting local initiatives between health education policy units and individual schools or authorities on the developing of HIV awareness in school children and young people. However, there was less evidence of organisational links with health authorities or social services. Few teachers were aware of DES guidelines on HIV/AIDS in schools, or how this related to their responsibilities in developing the curriculum in the area of personal and social education. Few opportunities were created in schools to discuss these issues with other professionals in the school setting – such as school doctors, nurses, education welfare officers – or to discuss how they, as teachers, could make a contribution to school policies. Policy guidance for staff working in special needs education was a particularly neglected area, and the difficulties of producing material or programmes that met a wide range of educational attainment or range requires highly motivated and specialist help and support. There was a dearth of information on how private schools and residential boarding schools or those with different religious denominations were responding to the needs of staff and children on HIV issues.

Positive policies – enhancing good childcare practices

Social services professionals in both the voluntary and statutory sectors reported similar experiences of the variation in organisational responses on policies. They stressed the difficulty of developing good childcare practice without coherent strategies. When agencies do have good policies and procedures for implementation this supports staff in carrying out their professional tasks and tends to encourage better relationships with consumer groups of parents and carers.

Poor resources

There was strong criticism of policies for children in care, which failed to provide a framework for offering them support, guidance and counselling on health and sex education, or on drug misuse, or in the development of social skills in preparation for leaving care. Staff working with vulnerable young people frequently mentioned the lack of organisational response to requests for resources and staff support.

Professional concerns

Professional priorities concerned the need to update their own knowledge on HIV in relation to modes of transmission in children, health and safety procedures, medical care and treatment protocols, and social/care planning.

Information needs

Experienced staff working with HIV positive children and parents were overwhelmed with requests to act as an information resource in research, medical treatment and training – often without any formal recognition of the additional burden this placed on staff time, resources and work schedules. Lack of professional confidence in their practice skills is understandably common, as few people have had any first hand experience, but sustained interest in HIV issues can be difficult as many people are still not sure whether there is a 'phoney war' situation relating to HIV in children. The gravity of the present and future circumstances need to be more widely disseminated, with *clear* presentation of statistics relating to HIV infection in the child population.

Paediatric staff identified the need to develop unified guidance on the medical management of HIV infection in children, which was still in a state of evolution by trial and error. Many of the comparisons between the progress of the disease in children in the UK and the USA were proving to be dissimilar in some aspects, making exchange of information and experience only partially useful. Making sense of the different medical approaches to a range of therapies, including treatment with powerful drugs, was difficult and until their efficacy has been evaluated and monitored over significant time scales, there can be no early resolution. Information about the long-term survival rates for children who survive the first year of life is still unknown – neither is it known with any certainty what the quality of their lives will be.

Staff felt that there was a need to share current medical information and experience with other colleagues, and suggested establishing a forum where ideas could be pooled and shared. Recently a group of paediatricians has begun meeting to act as such a forum, discussing experiences of treating children and addressing issues related to counselling parents on the care of their children, on bereavement, and on working with dying children.

Unreal expectations

In contrast, some staff felt that professional roles were expanding unrealistically to take on complex issues which needed specialist skills and knowledge that were beyond their competence. Those mentioned most often were counselling on safer sexual practices, safer drug misuse, interpersonal relationships, bereavement counselling and ethical issues. Where multidisciplinary teams existed it was easier to identify skilled help, but doctors could find themselves working, in isolation, in a haemophilia centre where they were expected to be clinician, marriage guidance counsellor and social worker. The skills most lacking were acknowledged as the ability to communicate with children of all ages and abilities in a language that they understood. Staff found it extremely diffcult to discuss with children how they felt about their own illness, or that of other siblings or their parents. They found it difficult to discuss their emotional and social needs.

Power sharing

A leading doctor caring for HIV infected people once said that the only experts in HIV disease were those who were infected. Professional attitudes have been influenced by consumer groups who stress their belief in remaining in control over their own lives despite their illness, and who challenge professional power that excludes them from decisions about care and treatment. Information is power, and sharing expertise with parents of children with HIV is recognised as an important element in encouraging models of shared care. Shared care embraces concepts of sharing expertise and knowledge with a range of staff and carers, so that different services offer a network of support for parents who may be ill themselves and need respite care or hospitalisation, but continuity of care is also guaranteed for families who prefer to care for children whenever possible – in cooperation with other key people in the child's life. Professional expertise is still limited and is dependent on gaining the confidence and trust of parents in monitoring their child's health and how they respond to treatment therapies.

Paediatric staff in Edinburgh have devised close working relationships with parents and foster parents, making regular home visits, seeing children in clinics and working with support groups. Social workers in a haemophilia centre have found that sharing information with family members can strengthen family functioning and facilitate communication between different family members who may previously have found it difficult to express their anxieties, fears and emotional pain. The Children Act enshrines this concept of shared power and partnership and seeks to give parents more power, as joint partners in assessing and planning for children with special needs in partnership with local authorities and health authorities.[51] The Hall Report stresses the importance of parental involvement and advocates parent-held records in child health services,[52] and the National Children's Bureau report, *Working for Children, Children's Services and the NHS Review* emphasises the need to listen to the voice of the consumer.[53]

Not all professionals, however, will find it easy to relinquish their autonomy and may need to develop skills in sharing knowledge and in communication. Some parents do not share this optimistic view of professionals' willingness to relinquish power – they have experienced traditional attitudes that demote their skills and knowledge as parents, and withold basic information about treatment or ignore parents' questions, fears and concerns. Some parents are worried that HIV is becoming over-professionalised and that, with the growth of specialist workers, parents will be made to feel even *more* inadequate and de-skilled. Parents would prefer to see the role of experts as valued *allies* in supporting the family network to maintain independent living in a normal environment for as long as possible.

10. Models of care and practice

There is a continuous quest for good models of care and practice, with an underlying, implicit hope that somewhere the 'perfect model' exists which can be replicated elsewhere. However, care models are evolved and developed in response to a variety of national and local needs – to provide services for different groups of people and problems. The study did identify, however, some key principles which are significant in determining the likely successful outcome of good practice, and these are listed below. The most important of these was *flexibility*. People valued services that could respond to a range of needs and be flexible to changing stages of difficulties, or could adapt and respond quickly in times of crisis. That is why many people wanted to see greater provision for flexible day care and drop-in-centres, sheltered housing and hostel accommodation, rehabilitation units for parents and children, informal nurseries and play groups, holiday and respite care, hospice care, special needs residential care, counselling services, out-reach work, fostering and adoption, and childminding.

There are common elements that seem crucial in developing good models of care and practice, whether it be in establishing a specialist unit such as a rehabilitation centre for parents and children, in developing a health education programme in local schools or in providing guidance on childcare policies for HIV services in a local authority.

The following checklist provides some useful indicators that seem to be central both in developing good models of care or in ensuring that care is improved. The checklist consists of essential policy elements:

- a consistent set of policies on HIV has been developed;
- has well-trained staff – and training policies;
- good ratio of staffing levels exist in relation to work needs;
- adequate funds and resources are provided;
- good management support and staff supervision is provided;
- staff moral is high;
- services are non-judgemental and non-stigmatising;
- good communication links exist, with support from local communities;
- openness and flexibility in working practices is encouraged;
- a multidisciplinary team approach and the pooling of professional expertise is favoured;
- there are regular staff meetings for reviewing and monitoring services;
- there is active participation, consultation and involvement of people affected by HIV;
- the philosophy of a 'bottom-up' rather than a top-down approach to planning and problem-solving is promoted;
- there is a clear allocation of work and key workers are appointed;
- a continuum of care is provided – working across agency boundaries;
- there is good written information, in plain language that people can understand;
- children's needs, feelings and rights are respected;
- there is good support from elected members and officers.

11. Resource issues – financial implications

The study found little evidence that agencies had developed any coherent financial strategies for funding services for children with HIV and most funding seemed to be allocated in an *ad hoc* way, without any assessment of needs. This is an area where central government has some power and control and could, given the political will, encourage improvement. Central government could, through its funding mechanism, request the agencies it funds to be more accountable, and demonstrate that they have taken into account the needs of women and children when allocating funds.

The survey revealed that staff working in health authorities were more likely to have adequate funds than those working in community services or in small voluntary organisations. There was, however, a marked difference in the distribution of funds in health care with less than 5 per cent allocated to community care – an area which includes services for drug misusers *and* health education programmes. Resources for women and children's services – such as in ante-natal care, paediatics and some haemophilia centres – were often considered totally inadequate to meet the high levels of need. Staff specifically wanted higher staffing levels in nursery care, counselling, and social work support, as well as better information systems and administrative support. Paradoxically, many of these centres have developed national reputations for pioneering services but have *still* found it difficult to convince local managers of their needs.

There was little evidence that District Health Authorities were anticipating future costs of treating children with ever more sophisticated therapies, or considering the financial implications of caring for ill children and parents over a longer time scale.

Department of Health earmarked HIV/AIDS funding to local authority social services departments has only recently been allocated, and at this stage it is difficult to predict how funding within departments will be apportioned. Initially it would seem that, in general, money has been allocated for staff training and policy development. Few departments, except in areas of well known need (such as Lothian and Hammersmith and Fulham), have developed any comprehensive childcare services for infected children and families. There was little mention in the study of funding allocations to children with special needs or disabilities.

It was unclear from the study whether Local Education Authorities had identified specific allocation of funds for in-service training for teachers on HIV or for the development of the school curriculum in the field of personal and social education. Money *had* been allocated for appointing Drugs Coordinators in LEAs to develop HIV awareness in schools, but how these related to general strategies on HIV was uncertain. Some of this work is currently being evaluated, but there was little information about resources in individual schools, and it is not clear how head teachers and school governors will respond to HIV when they manage their own budgets under local management of schools.

The loudest complaints about funding came from the voluntary sector where it was felt that, in relation to the amount of pioneering work they were doing in work with children and young people, they were *grossly* under-resourced. They always felt financially vulnerable and were unable to make long-term plans when constantly faced with problems about survival. The smaller agencies felt that even when needs had been clearly established it was often dificult persuading statutory bodies to recognise their work. These were most likely to be agencies working with disadvantaged groups of young people – in street agencies, drugs services or the homeless. Many of these services call for high staffing ratios but, because of difficulties of measuring the effectiveness of preventative work, it could be hard to justify additional funding. Organisations catering for women and children also felt that they were less likely to attract funds because they tended to have a less powerful national voice in lobbying for resources.

Some national voluntary organisations were similarly grossly under-resourced in relation to the demands on their services. The Haemophilia Society is one such organisation. It is currently engaged in providing a range of services, including help in processing litigation and compensation for haemophiliacs infected with Factor VIII, establishing networks of local regional support groups, providing an information advice service, as well as campaiging for improved medical care and treatment. Yet it feels unable to develop many services – including specific work on children's needs – because of inadequate levels of staffing and a lack of financial resources. Criteria for funding the voluntary sector varied so much between different agencies and charities, that some staff found they spent much of their time writing different applications for finances – time which they felt was largely wasted.

Voluntary organisations and statutory bodies identified the growing problems of inadequate welfare benefits allocated to children and parents with HIV. These families often needed additional financial help in the form of diet, clothing, transport and carers' allowances. There were many examples of families applying to the Social Fund for grants, particularly families with haemophilia. Problems of emergency funds for one-off payments was also frequently mentioned. Statistics collated by the Haemophilia Society showed a high level of young people with HIV were dependent on social security benefits.

The following checklist of questions could be helpful in considering allocation of resources by different agencies, whether in the health, education or social services:

- Do financial strategies on HIV indicate specific allocation of budgets for the development of services for children and parents? Do they specify what they are? For example:
  - ante-natal care;
  - paediatric services;
  - training foster parents;
  - respite care;
  - drug services;
  - needle exchange;
  - community centre;
  - training staff;
  - health education;
  - day nurseries, playgroups.
- What priority ranking do they have?
- What criteria are used in assessing financial needs?

- Have staff/consumer groups been consulted in drawing up budgets?
- Have resources been allocated for children with special needs?
- Do funding agencies have clear criteria for funding voluntary organisations, and are they consulted in drawing up HIV strategies?
- How do agencies monitor the financial impact of HIV disease in families? Do they conduct research into issues of welfare benefits and payments, including research on the effects on health care of inadequate DSS payments?
- Do any local agencies provide emergency funding for people in financial crises?
- In areas where many agencies have HIV subgroups is there co-ordinating machinery for rationalising funding allocations, such as joint consultative committees, or are there other mechanisms?
- What resources are allocated for housing needs, welfare rights, advice for families and children with HIV?

12. Black and minority ethnic issues

The study identified the need to develop appropriate community-based services for Black and minority ethnic communities and to adopt non-discriminatory and anti-racist policies, which also address religious and cultural diversities.

It was considered that there is a need to appoint more staff recruited from Black and minority ethnic communities in children and family services. There is also a need to appoint hospital and community-based link workers and translators who can also act as skilled advocates. There needs to be provision of information, posters and leaflets including audio and video material and education packages on HIV/AIDS in minority languages.

The survey revealed that there was a small but significant number of HIV positive women and children from Black and minority ethnic groups who were mainly located in the Thames region and had special needs because of their social situation. Although they had come from many different parts of the African continent, Asia and the Middle East these people shared some common problems. The parent was usually herself HIV positive and had most probably acquired HIV infection in her country of origin, from heterosexual activity, blood transfusions or drug misuse. In one ante-natal clinic in London, a third of all women diagnosed as HIV positive had come from overseas.[54] A typical profile of these women tended to be that they were living alone, some having been deserted by their husband/partner when they learned of their HIV status. They may have come here to study or work and were not aware of their HIV infection at the time. They were often living alone in poor, rented accommodation or were homeless and living in Part 3 accommodation. They were terrified that someone might learn about their status and tell family members, and some were too afraid to return home – fearing rejection, shame and stigma. For these reasons they were sometimes more reluctant to talk to someone from their own culture, fearing breaches of confidentiality. They may not speak English and so find it difficult to understand information about treatment therapies or how to apply for social work help and support. Some parents refuse to send children to school in case the teachers find out. One parent was so paranoid that she changed the children's schooling *seven* times. In addition, some families are engaged in lengthy legal wrangles with immigration authorities over their refugee status or over residential permits. Some mothers have become too ill to care for their children and, even when they are terminally ill, have refused to make long-term care plans for their surviving children.

All of these difficulties create special problems in caring for children and parents. Their needs can only be adequately met by adopting policies that promote more ethnically sensitive services and by training staff in all settings to develop awareness of these issues and to build up better links and resources within the Black and ethnic communities – links through which we can begin to address problems of alienation and isolation. Particular attention to the needs of young Black children in care – who are over-represented as a percentage of all children in care – must be paid so that they do not experience additional racial prejudice and stereotyping in relation to HIV issues.

Recommendations

- HIV Policies for children and families must include the provision of services that meet the needs of Black and minority ethnic groups. They must also develop services which reach out to isolated families.
- Agencies should appoint staff who are recruited from Black and minority ethnic communities who are trained in providing appropriate services which meet the needs of people, irrespective of language, religious and cultural diversities.
- Agencies should recruit and train foster parents and adopters from Black and minority ethnic communities.
- Organisations from minority communities are able to encourage channels of communication about HIV issues and should be seen as a resource by agencies for forging links with different

communities and for assisting in the building of local networks of support services.

- Special attention may need to be paid to the social, educational and health care needs of children, who may face particular problems of social isolation, may be missing educational opportunities, and may have few opportunities to mix with children of their own age.

13. Ethical and legal problems

There are a number of policies which should be clarified in relation to legal and ethical issues which affect all aspects of work on HIV and affected children's needs. These cover the following:

- HIV and testing procedures and policies;
- confidentiality;
- informed consent – the age of consent and consent to treatment;
- policies in fostering and adoption;
- sex education and health education;
- caring for children;
- rights of children;
- monitoring HIV – role of Ethical Committees and advisory groups;
- discrimination.

Many of the legal and ethical questions raised in HIV related work have been the subject of detailed guidance from professional bodies and trade unions, and from government circulars and directives. Some organisations have issued written policies which explicitly describe procedures governing the limitations and boundaries of practice, but more commonly there is sparse knowledge and understanding of some of the issues raised – and there are few sanctions to invoke if legal and ethical boundaries are crossed.

Importantly, the problem arises with children because their views are more likely to be ignored or over-ruled by adults, who are in a more powerful position. Children in care often have no idea what their rights are, or whether or not they can withhold consent – either for medical treatment or for being tested for HIV infection. Similarly, they rarely have any control over who has access to confidential information, and many children are subjected to humiliation, ostracism and punishment if it becomes known that they have been 'exposed' to situations which have increased the risk of them contracting HIV infection.

Young people of 16 years or over should never be tested without their informed consent, and this implies that full counselling is available to them so that they understand what is involved. But the situation arises quite frequently in residential care where staff are neither properly trained, or aware of the legal and ethical issues involved in the concept of informed consent. In these cases children are not genuinely consulted and formal procedures to guide staff in this area are usually non-existent.

Childcare organisations such as British Agencies for Adoption and Fostering (BAAF) do not advise that children being considered for fostering or adoption should be tested for HIV infection.[55] This is justified on several counts, for example, because the test is unreliable under two years of age, and also because it would not be either desirable or ethically sound to screen all children without implicitly acknowledging that the test in young children reveals the HIV status of the mother – and without her informed consent, the test would breach *her* privacy and rights. Only if a mother gives her informed consent should a decision be taken on whether to proceed or not with the test. The authority of the Local Authority to reveal information about the HIV status of a child, without the consent of the parent, remains unclear. It will no doubt at some point be tested through legal proceedings. Most organisations need to be clearer about the ethics of testing. In Hammersmith and Fulham they believe that children and young people in statutory care can only be considered for testing 'if there is evidence that the health care and management of the child will be adversely affected without the test being done. It will not be considered on the grounds of sexuality and lifestyle of the child, young person or parent(s) alone'.

Clearly issues of testing, care and treatment of children raise important questions of principle about how much children understand and whether they are expected to have their views listened to. With children under the age of 16 years a doctor must still judge whether the child is competent to consent to the test on his or her behalf. If the doctor's answer is yes then the child's consent must be sought, according to the General Medical Council (GMC) guidance.[56] In those cases where it is deemed to be in the child's interest to override the wishes of parents, such as in parental sexual abuse, the competent child can give *informed* consent, although normally the consent of parents, or local authorities who are *in loco parentis,* should be obtained.

The ethical issues facing staff involved in developing awareness about health education and prevention of infection in relation to sexual behaviour, sex education and drug misuse are especially difficult – and are fraught with contradictions. Recent legislation makes it difficult for teachers to talk about sex and sexuality if by doing so they appear to be 'promoting' homosexuality – a dictum which is enshrined in Section 28 of The Local Government Act 1988. This states that a Local Authority shall not:

'(a) intentionally promote homosexuality or publish material with the intention of promoting homosexuality.

(b) promote teaching in any maintained school of the acceptability of homosexuality as a pretended family relationship.

(c) Nothing in sub section (1) above shall be taken to prohibit the doing of anything for the purpose of treating or preventing the spread of disease.'

So public health campaigns and government policies are urging young people to be sexually more responsible, and yet are withholding the means whereby young people can discuss and explore their own sexuality in an informed and structured setting – in the learning environment of a school.

Experienced educators such as HMI's in their document *Health Education from Five to Sixteen* advocate honest, objective and open discussion in sex education programmes, including issues of homosexuality, contraception, sexually transmitted diseases and abortion.[57]

Staff caring for children in residential care and schools also face difficult legal and ethical problems if they hand out free condoms or suggest how to practice safer sex to children below the legal age of consent for sexual intercourse. Staff caring for over 16s can be in difficulty if they appear to endorse an acknowledgement of a young person's sexuality or appear to be tacitly encouraging them in their sexual behaviour. These contradictions clearly confront the hypocrisy and double standards that surround attitudes to children and young people. Often children are in care because they may have experienced sexual abuse and violence from an early age. They may well be sexually experienced but emotionally very damaged and in need of skilled and knowledgeable counselling so that anxieties, fears and distorted perceptions in their understanding of sexual behaviour, and relationships can be explored within the context of a supportive environment.

Children with special educational needs raise important problems about how best to communicate and educate them about their rights concerning testing, consent to treatment, and their right to have a sexual life. Despite some advances in accepting that children with learning difficulties should be able to live more integrated lives in the community, staff and parents continue to find it difficult to know how best to prepare young people and children in areas of personal choice such as sexual behaviour or drug misuse. Denial about what children and young people with special needs really want or how they actually behave is still a powerful factor. A small survey of the understanding of HIV issues held by residents in a long-stay hospital illustrated this vividly, where accounts of residents' views on HIV were either very explicit or misinformed. The residents also continued, despite the restrictions of institutional life, to have a rich and secret sex life.[58]

Tackling these problems ethically and honestly will require highly trained staff who are committed to wanting to bring about a better quality life for this group of children.

In order to protect patients and consumers of services, there is a need to monitor policies. Professional staff need to be clear about informing consumers of their rights. Some local authorities have established Ethical Committees, with representation from consumers, whose role is to monitor all aspects of HIV services in the authority.

Recommendations

- Agency policies should provide detailed guidance covering legal and ethical procedures. Guidance should be published and available to all consumers and staff.
- Staff support, training and access to expert legal advice should be available to all staff working with young people.
- Children in care should have access to independent counselling advice on issues relating to testing and consent to treatment. They should be informed of their legal rights in respect of laws relating to sex, such as, the age of majority, the age of consent to sexual

intercourse, contraception and abortion, homosexuality, rape and indecent exposure.

- Staff need specialist training on communicating with children about health education and preventative health, particularly in areas related to safer sex and drug use, sex and sexuality.
- Agencies should establish Ethics Committees and monitor ethical problems.

Part III

14. The USA experience

The substance of this chapter is based on research of HIV and AIDS undertaken in the USA. A list of projects and visits of observation made to programmes in the USA on treatment and care of children and families with HIV and AIDS appears at the end of the chapter.

The size and scale of the problem of HIV infection in children and women is on a very different level, so making comparisons may not be all that helpful. In New York State alone 1,000 babies with HIV infection had been born to infected women by 1988. (AIDS is now the leading cause of death among women aged 25–40 in New York City.)[59] The statistics for the states of Florida and New Jersey are not far behind. It is estimated that by 1991 there will be between 10,000 and 20,000 babies infected with HIV in New York State. Ninety per cent are born to Black and Hispanic women, 90 per cent of families are on welfare and 60 per cent of children are cared for by extended families, foster parents or adoptive parents. Forty per cent are born to single parents who are in their teens or early twenties. However, the majority of babies with HIV are born to women with a drug using problem or who are the sexual partners of a drug user. Many women do not realise they are HIV positive until they become pregnant. Because many children are born to women who already have symptomatic HIV infection the children are likely to manifest more severe symptoms, earlier, resulting in terminal illness.

This preponderance of more severely infected children has shaped the direction of services in the USA. Children are more likely to show signs of developmental delays, motor and neurological impairment including speech delays, hearing and vision loss, as well as more non-specific symptoms such as failure to thrive. Many of the programmes

visited have, therefore, concentrated on early educational intervention – with strong emphasis on a range of therapies to counteract the
impact of long bouts of hospitalisation, lack of emotional stimulus
and the impact of social isolation on social and cognitive skills.

Much greater emphasis is placed on psycho-social therapeutic
work with ill children and support for families. The impact on
families is also devastating, and a new phenomenon – that of
abandoning HIV infected babies in hospitals – has led to the
establishment of substitute care by volunteer older women from
similar ethnic backgrounds who have been encouraged to provide a
volunteer 'granny' programme. These schemes involve senior
citizens who are paid a small fee to visit and befriend one or two
children in the hospital and develop a caring relationship with them.
Some of these schemes have led to subsequent foster care placements. Finding and recruiting foster families has obviously been a
great problem and it is still difficult to recruit and train enough high
calibre people who are willing to take on the onerous task and
emotional stress of caring for one or two very ill children.

South Florida has been particularly overwhelmed with the
number of children in need of foster care. In the three counties of
Dade, Broward and Palm Beach, there are 860 HIV infected children
under three years of age who need long-term fostering. Many of them
are suffering from birth defects compounded by the use of drugs
such as crack by their parents during pregnancy. One centre has
specialised in developing intensive support work with parents and
children. It has introduced a baby 'buddy' scheme, where a
volunteer visits the home and works with the child and parent to
encourage and stimulate the child's emotional, educational and
social development. At the same time, another worker works in
supporting the parent. This home visiting scheme supplements
provision at a family-based day care centre for parents and children
who meet regularly for help and advice on medical and social issues.

In Newark, New Jersey, the United Hospital is one of the leading
paediatric HIV/AIDS treatment centres in the USA. At its Friday
morning clinic it treats up to 70 children, ranging in age from young
babies to 16-year-olds. It has a highly organised and impressive
multidisciplinary team of immunologists, paediatricians, paediatric
nurses, dieticians, speech therapists, social workers, neurologists
and physiotherapists. A weekly team meeting is held and reviews
current treatment goals, identifies social and emotional needs, and

allocates tasks to key workers. The relationship between professionals appears to be open and non-hierarchical and the staff all make valuable contributions to the final outcome of the case conference.

The children treated at the clinic are often undergoing stressful and painful medical interventions and their social and medical problems are very complex. Whilst professional staff are interviewing children and their parents there are key volunteers, who work closely with clinical staff, to help families. This voluntary help includes sometimes transporting families to the clinics, playing with children in activities rooms, or remaining with children undergoing lengthy out-patient treatment – some of them can be there for four or five hours. They also liaise closely with social workers in linking with the home environment.

Here are some examples of the problems faced by children and their carers which are presented at the weekly case review – the situations have been changed to respect confidentiality.

A three-year-old child was rushed into the hospital. He has HIV infection, has a drug abusing mother and has twice swallowed his mother's drugs.

An eight-year-old – his mother died a month ago from AIDS and he has been placed with temporary foster parents. The child is grieving badly for his mother, exacerbated by cultural difficulties. The child is Black and has been placed with Hispanic foster parents. He is having a hard time adjusting to a very different diet. The foster parents don't have much money and they need a prescription for vitamins. It is agreed the social worker will visit and talk to the foster parents about the diet and explore what can be done with him in play therapy about his grieving.

A four-year-old – is having problems digesting his food and is vomiting after each meal. There is concern to try to stabilise his weight loss, and a dietician will discuss this and advise parents.

A 16-year-old – with haemophilia and AIDS. It is his first visit to the hospital. His T Helper count is down. The family are in crisis because of his condition and need a great deal of help and support. He will have to be hospitalised for at least two weeks.

A 15-year-old-girl – has gained weight but is refusing to take AZT. She is very depressed and has made two previous attempts at suicide. She has an injecting drug user boyfriend and has been prostituting. She has been referred to the adolescent services for counselling.

A six-year-old – has herpes, Lymphocytic Interstitial Pneumonia (LIP), chronic oral thrush, asthma. He is on gamma globulin, but his appetite is good. He is attending school regularly and family morale is good.

Across the road from the hospital the first day care nursery unit for children with HIV has recently been opened. It takes up to 30 children daily. The children are collected in a mini-bus from their homes each day, enabling their parents, who are often sick themselves, to have a rest. The nursery is staffed by trained teachers, nurses, carers and volunteers. A social worker liaises with the parents and ensures that problems of diet, treatment, transport and welfare payments are resolved. The nursery was established because these children were not accepted at other day nurseries – provision of day care for the under fives is difficult to obtain in New York State.

The programme at the day nursery considers the *total* needs of the child, and places an emphasis on early education and developmental stimulus. The staff have noticed a marked improvement in some children since they enrolled. Neurological impairment and physical and mental delays are common, and children are carefully assessed and monitored weekly, with careful charts being kept to record progress. Children are lavishly praised when they pass small but important milestones of improvement.

At the Van Etten Hospital in the Bronx, a paediatric AIDS day care centre provides an intensive but relaxed programme of day care with nursery and pre-school education for up to 25 children. This number is broken down into two groups of infant and toddlers (six months to three years) and pre-school (children of three years and over). The team includes seven teachers, a social worker, a nurse, dietary aides, bus drivers and escorts, who also act as aides in the classroom. It has its own mini-bus used for transporting children and for providing special outings.

Most children are with foster parents or with adoptive parents, with only a few of the children living with their natural families. The centre offers children an enhanced early childhood education which seeks to compensate for disturbed early childhood experience, emotional traumas and separation, and problems which arise from the effects of HIV disease on physical and emotional development. Child psychiatric services support children in coping with terminal illness and helping children to express their feelings. The service also helps staff to cope with their feelings and with the stress they experience in working with very sick children.

The third 'arm' of the centre is the development of a support service for children and their families. Social workers liaise with the families who meet regularly for support. The emphasis is on integrating families into the day centre where they can learn about their child's experience and take pleasure in being part of the philosophy of encouraging, learning about normal learning and growth.

The medical staff liaise closely with the centre, but because some medical procedures are painful and frightening, these treatments are performed elsewhere. The aim is to keep the day centre as a safe place emotionally for children to experience how to play and learn together.

Conclusion

In a workshop on HIV Children and Parents convened by the USA Surgeon General in 1987, experts drawn from health, education and welfare services called repeatedly for comprehensive, coordinated and accessible health, welfare, social and financial services for children and parents infected by HIV.[60] Since then the incidence and spread of HIV infection in children and parents has increased alarmingly. The most valuable lesson to be drawn from any visit to the USA is to witness the outcome of 'diswelfare', and to sit in any busy clinic and listen to the personal case histories of families struggling to survive against overwhelming obstacles of poverty in obtaining even basic health and welfare care. Preventing the spread of HIV infection in children and parents in the UK will need continual vigilance and vigorous commitment by Government to well-funded and comprehensive, free, national health services and social care programmes which are both accessible and non-discriminatory and do not impose any financial or legal restrictions on access. Any policies which tend to destabilise the universal provision of decent health and social care may severely undermine future provision of HIV services. Experience of the USA problems remains as a serious warning.

There are, however, also many valuable lessons that can be learnt from the USA experience which are relevant for UK experiences. Some of these are briefly mentioned below. The work of the multidisciplinary team in Newark has stressed the complexity of the problems and the importance of providing coordinated and comprehensive care for all family members. Some of the issues faced in the American experience provide valuable insights which can be used to re-evaluate the approaches to childcare services in the UK.

- There is provision of better written information in simple language – attractively produced in booklet form with illustrations – for families and carers. The tone used is friendly, straightforward and non-patronising.
- There is greater emphasis on early childhood stimulation, paralleled by encouraging the parenting and educational skills of parents themselves – allowing them to be involved and helping them to enlarge their own skills in caring for their children.
- The use of volunteers is more widespread in work with children in hospital, day care settings and home visiting schemes. Many children have their own 'buddy volunteer'. This recognises that children are often as needy as their parents, and both require a great deal of individual care and attention.
- There is great attention paid to providing psycho-social and therapeutic help for children in hospital settings and the development of adolescent counselling for children.
- The multidisciplinary team approach recognises the value and complementary nature of specialists such as dieticians, nutritionists, speech therapists.
- Many States and counties in the USA have established 'AIDS Review Panels for Children'. These panels establish policy on all issues relating to children in care and develop criteria for fostering, adoption, treatment, schooling, testing, and so on.
- There are national organisations which are developing and stimulating discussion and policies on a range of issues. The Paediatric AIDS Coalition monitors and lobbies for legislation. The Children's AIDS Task Force develops and encourages position papers, and policies on all aspects of the problem.

USA visits

Visits of observation were made to the following programmes in the USA.

- Centre One Project Simulation
  Ft Lauderdale
  Florida
- Human Resource Services
  Dade County
  Florida

- Dr Tuemala
  Obstetrician
  Brigham Women's Hospital
  Boston
- Dr Lynn Mofenson
  Division of Communicable Disease Control
  Massachusetts Department of Health
  Boston
- Human Resource Services
  Boston
  Foster Placement Team
- Dr Margaret Heagarty
  Harlem Hospital
  New York
- Susan Wojtasike
  Child Life Director
  Belle Vue Hospital
  New York
- Caroline Lelyveld
  Day Care Centre Van Etten Hospital
  Bronx
  New York
- Ayre Rubenstein
  Albert Einstein College of Medicine
  Bronx
  New York
- Mary Boland and Dr James Oleske
  United Hospital
  Newark
  New Jersey
- Babyland
  Day Care Centre
  Newark
  New Jersey

15. Summary and recommendations

This book opened by providing an overview of the main issues raised by this study. In this summary, suggestions are made about key areas for further work and attention is drawn to the main recommendations for future action. A more detailed set of recommendations arising from the survey appears in Appendix 2.

Marginalisation of children's needs
The overriding concern emerging from this report is the continuation of cultural and organisational norms which marginalise children's needs and concerns. Current preoccupation with managing change in health, education and social services will tend to reinforce this marginalisation in relation to HIV services for children, unless the opportunity is used to integrate HIV services into mainstream provision. Putting the needs of children first and providing child-centred services is of paramount importance. Legitimising children's views and feelings can foster the development of self-esteem, responsibility and maturity in handling future difficulties and personal traumas. But changing professional attitudes, retraining staff and adopting service goals which re-orientate philosophies is not easy. It will require new approaches which are non-hierarchical and see children and their parents as equal partners in combating HIV disease. It requires far more attention to be paid in developing age-related information and educational programmes, clear and jargon-free advice on care and treatment, and access to independent counselling on all aspects of HIV concerns. This review of childcare needs in relation to HIV disease has merely served to highlight areas of neglect and underdevelopment in many areas of childcare practice. Overcoming barriers to change takes time but it is

vital, in the interests of children, that services begin to review their practice and actively promote the development of a more child-centred environment – as a matter of urgency.

Drug misuse and HIV

Attention on the needs of children at risk born to HIV infected parents in Scotland has been intense over the last few years and has attracted national media coverage, research studies and intense professional interests. It is surprising therefore to realise that, despite this 'glasshouse' attention, services are not that well developed, resourced or integrated on the ground, and many of the key services for children and drug misusing families are struggling to survive – even though they are pioneering new ways of working with children, families and carers. In particular, services for families with drug related problems are still incoherent and fragmented. Paradoxically, despite concentrated media attention on the Scottish dimension of HIV disease, policy makers elsewhere have been reluctant to recognise or develop drug services for families and have ignored the evidence of increased HIV transmission in injecting drug use – throughout the UK.

Haemophilia and HIV

It is worrying that the single largest group of children diagnosed as being HIV positive, that is haemophiliac boys, has merited so little special attention or serious studies of their needs and concerns. There have been studies examining the progression of HIV disease in children and accounts of problems associated with counselling families and adolescents, but their problems are complex and on-going, and the study indicates that there is undoubtedly a residue of related difficulties and problems for school children which may be dealt with very inadequately. Fear of exposing their children to stigma and isolation has reinforced family isolation but this understandable need for privacy should not totally override the need to facilitate helping children to express their concerns and give them an opportunity to share what has been experienced. It should be possible to explore with haemophilia organisations and parent groups how to approach undertaking such a study.

Minority ethnic issues

There is a reluctance to discuss publicly the increased numbers of children infected with HIV from minority ethnic communities who are being treated in the Greater London region. This is understandable as there is concern about reinforcing racialist stereotyping about HIV disease. But these families do present a challenge to all agencies to provide improved services which are more ethnically sensitive. The provision of services which reflect cultural, religious and language differences is still underdeveloped and there is a need to engage in more effective discussion with different minority ethnic communities so that realistic appraisal of support networks can be established. From this discussion process more effective multicultural resources can, and should, be developed.

The education system and HIV

It is difficult to address the needs of vulnerable groups of children such as those with learning difficulties, special needs or disabilities, in relation to HIV issues, often because of strong feelings of overprotection, and emotional barriers of denial and panic affecting both staff and parents. Parents, children and staff need effective educational materials and skilled communicators in supporting them to develop HIV policies in school settings and residential establishments. Some work has been developed in looking at the needs of children with learning difficulties, but there is still considerable work needed to develop effective strategies for a range of children with special needs.

Children in the private sector

Little is known about the standard of care or whether HIV policies have been developed in the private sector of education and residential care for children. Some private boarding schools have acknowledged that it is an important issue but are often not aware of where to look for guidance. Education authorities should ensure that all private schools registered in its area are informed about HIV issues and encouraged to develop their own policies. Schools should have access to local education authority resources for advice and information if they require help.

Communicating with children

All professional groups acknowledged their lack of knowledge and experience of the communication skills and techniques needed in face to face work with children. In the long-term these problems have to be addressed in professional course curriculum training but, in the short term, professional associations, employees and training bodies should provide short-term post-graduate courses and in-service training.

Children in care

Protecting the rights of children in care is essential. They should be given all relevant information on local authority HIV policies and access to independent counselling and advice on HIV testing, treatment and care plans. Their views and feelings should be formally recorded in any decision-making about their welfare. Children will need appropriate, age-related information material on how to manage their illness and how to take care of themselves.

Equally relevant here are the comments about improving staff training in both the long and short term (*see* above).

Sharing power with families

Families and foster parents expressed strong views about the need for professionals to treat them as equal partners in sharing the care of HIV children. They wanted to be consulted and informed about treatment, and to have their views listened to and respected. Parents were often more skilled and experienced in day-to-day management of the children (and their condition) than professional staff, and this should be recognised. Information and advice was a two-way process. Parents felt that they need better information, written in simple user friendly language, which would help them in caring for themselves and their children. A strong preference for family-centred primary care treatment centres, staffed by multidisciplinary teams was expressed. It was generally felt that such centres are more likely to meet the needs of the whole family unit – with the health of children and parents being monitored together and the family's health needs being viewed as a whole.

The response to HIV infection in children

The lack of government response in promoting the development of HIV services for children is both regrettable and very worrying. It is still puzzling to conjecture why the known cumulative numbers of over 894 children and young people (aged 0–19 years) with HIV has aroused so little debate in comparison to the strong professional lobbies mounted at the beginning of HIV infection in adults in the UK. The Social Services Committee called for further research into the needs of children (the Seventh HIV/AIDS Report and Select Committee on Social Services) and this mapping exercise suggested that, even where there are known clusters of children with HIV, there is a reluctance to develop a coherent response. Typically, HIV issues specifically related to women and children tend to have been 'tagged on' almost as an afterthought when viewing the problems of HIV in general – even in districts where figures of affected women and children are already significant.

A national forum on HIV and children

This lack of coherent response may be partially attributed to the fact that there is no national voice cogently representing the particular needs of children who are HIV positive. Many parents fear exposure for themselves and their children, as has been demonstrated by the work and experiences of organisations such as Positively Women and the Haemophilia Society. Even childcare organisations in the voluntary sector have experienced difficulties in persuading their member organisations to take a more proactive stance on HIV related issues and are often concerned that HIV issues still remain marginalised.

There is undoubtedly a need to establish a national forum for bringing together relevant organisations, professional groups and users of services who can campaign for a more effective provision, undertake further research, and act as a forum for exchange and dissemination of information on all aspects of medical care and treatments and social care. The National Children's Bureau already has a role in bringing together a wide range of childcare interest in the voluntary and statutory sector, and this organisation is in the best position to explore such developments – and to encourage wider debate amongst its constituents. This could take the form of a standing committee on HIV in Children and Families and its role could include responsibility for up-to-date information, conducting research, commissioning the publication of educational materials, reviewing and monitoring developments in treatment, services, policies and funding.

Recommendations

- Research should be commissioned concerning the collation of data on children with HIV. Such research should aim to refine present categories, as defined by CDSC, in order to develop a more accurate picture. (See Chapter 2.)
- Services for women should be coordinated so that a continuum of care is offered, and the health of HIV women and their children are considered within a family-centred service. (See Chapter 3.)
- Family profiles are different. Services should respond to differing needs, recognising diversity by offering a flexible approach which is non-judgemental and non-discriminatory. (See Chapter 4.)
- Central Government should issue guidelines on HIV childcare issues to relevant statutory departments. It should require Local Authorities and District Health Authorities to develop specific strategic planning for services for children with HIV. Government should also ensure that this is adequately financed, through its funding mechanism. (See Chapter 5.)
- Children's rights and needs have been neglected and, as a matter of priority, all services should now develop a child-centred approach. It must be acknowledged that communicating with children is important. Children should have access to independent counselling services, and age-appropriate written information and educational material. (See Chapter 6.)
- There is a need to develop more simple user-friendly information for children and families. This must include translation of materials into minority ethnic languages. (See Chapter 6.)
- Voluntary organisations have a crucial role in promoting the needs of HIV children and families. They should act to stimulate developing work with children with special needs, to conduct research and to promote the welfare of children in residential care. (See Chapter 7.)
- All staff working with children need to undertake in-service training on HIV issues. There is a need to develop specialist modules on communication skills. Training should be provided for *all* carers and volunteers. (See Chapter 8.)
- Professional and organisational issues hinder the development of integrated services – it must be recognised that the sharing of power with the users of services is important. (See Chapter 9.)

- Models of Good Practice – the provision of a checklist of key elements in developing good practice is suggested. (See Chapter 10.)
- Resources should be allocated for HIV services for children, and priorities should be agreed. (See Chapter 11.)
- Minority ethnic communities have needs which are not fully recognised and these must be addressed. This includes the training and recruitment of minority ethnic staff and developing ethnically sensitive material. This should take account of language, religious and cultural diversity, and adopt non-discriminatory and anti-racist policies. (See Chapter 12.)
- The legal and ethical issues for children and families are often ignored. All organisations should issue guidance on legal and ethical procedures. (See Chapter 13.)
- There is a need to develop coherent and integrated HIV policies for children bringing together health, education and social services in each locality. (See Chapter 15.)
- A Standing Conference on HIV and Childcare Issues should be established as a national forum for promoting the welfare of children, young people and their families, for disseminating and exchanging information, and for conducting research. (See Chapter 15.)

16. Letters and poems
from Brenda House

When I was 16-years-old, I was having my son, who is now three. I was in labour, about to have the baby, and one of the doctors mentioned my baby's father had taken drugs. They phoned his doctor and found out he had HIV.

At the same time they told me my baby would not be allowed in the nursery, and I would not be allowed to walk up and down the hospital or go to the TV room. After having the baby, I was wheeled back to my room in a gown covered in blood. I was in for ten days. My room didn't get cleaned, my dishes were always left there all day and my blood stained sheets were hardly ever changed, as the nurses tried as hard as possible to avoid my room.

I was stuck in a horrible little room at the end of the ward, away from mothers with new babies. I had a bathroom next door to me, with a 'Danger of Infection' sticker on it. I was offered no support from the nurses, only rejection – all of which made me feel bitter about the treatment I had received.

This all happened in 1986, and it's now 1989, and I believe that people are still treated the same way. It's sad to believe that the so-called 'caring profession' can be so uncaring and ignorant.

August 1989

I found out I was HIV Positive in February 1987, after the death of my husband. We had obviously had it for a few years, because we had stopped using IV drugs years ago. We thought we had missed it, and how lucky we were!

My health had not been very good, but when he died, I went downhill fast.

In August 1988, I was feeling very weak and had a bad bout of flu, so I called the doctor to come and see me. The doctor came and gave me a prescription for antibiotics. I could not collect this medication, as I felt too weak to walk down town to the chemist. In the afternoon I felt so weak, I crawled to the toilet. I started haemorrhaging – I had never seen so much blood in my life. I was frightened, so I called the doctor to ask advice, and what was happening to me.

She told me that this can happen to people when they are unwell, and not to worry. This was on a Friday, and she said to phone over the weekend if things got worse. They did, I phoned, and the doctor said I would not bleed to death over the weekend, and to phone back on Monday. I could not raise the energy to argue.

I was slipping in and out of consciousness, but kept going. I phoned on Monday and spoke to my own GP, who came right away. He got a shock when he saw me – he had to climb in the window, as I could not get up. He phoned the local hospital. When he mentioned HIV, they said they would not take me. He phoned several hospitals, all to no avail, because of HIV. He got back on the local hospital again and said 'Look, this woman needs blood now, or she will die!'

An ambulance came for me, and the drivers were told not to touch me. When I arrived at the hospital, it was like spacemen coming to meet me.

I was put in a room, and no one was allowed in, it had a big sign on the door – 'DO NOT ENTER – HIGH RISK!'

The doctor came to take a blood sample to measure my blood count, in order to work out how much blood I would need. He was covered from head to toe, and had plastic goggles on his eyes. There was no communication, he looked at me as if I was some vile creature, the pits of the earth.

I wanted to die – he made me feel so horrible – words cannot describe it. In all, I was given six units of blood, and hardly any food, as I think most of the nurses were too afraid to come into my room.

I was not allowed to use a toilet, I had to use cardboard bedpans. They gave me a bottle of liquid called ASEPT and told me to pour some into the urine, and it was to be left for one hour, and then someone would get rid of it. No-one came to remove any urine from my room, and so there were lots of full bedpans lying around. There were to be no cleaners in my room, and my linen was only changed once in ten days, when it was very soiled. In those conditions who could eat anyway – even if I had been given a meal.

There were to be no kind words. Even a smile would have done, but alas no. As far as they were concerned, I was just a walking deadly germ that did not need any – or rather did not deserve any – humane treatment.

I had two visitors, they were made to wear gowns, gloves, hats, etc., and were made to feel so embarrassed about even knowing me, it was too much for them to come back.

I was given hormone tablets to try and stop the bleeding. When it had stopped for 18 hours, they told me I was to go home. I asked why all this bleeding had occurred, they said they did not know, and if I had any further trouble, to go to a hospital in Edinburgh.

I was just so relieved to be getting out of that room which I had been in for fourteen days, and away from those under-educated, unfeeling people, who call themselves professionals. I went without so much as, 'well, it could have been this or that' – no explanation at all. Just, 'We don't know and we don't want to know, just don't come back'.

I won't!

August 1989

HIV you must be jokin'
I tell you man, I was boakin'
T cells and fours and 53s
It means nothing to someone like me
Tell me now will I die
Well we have this brand new drug to try
Would you like it now?
Would you like it later?
When you're being sick an' shittin' through a grater
When you're face gets thin and your eyes get big
When your hair falls out, you get an NHS wig
Gee, thats great, love the colour
You look 20 years older than your mother
Eat well, eat good they say
On fuckin' what, 10p a day?
I'm on income support you see
So they don't care about people like me
YOU'LL DIE

August 1989

Some People think the Arc I've got
Is similar to Noah's cot
They think its just for animals see
They've never stopped to look at me

All they see is my disease
Have another look now please
She's a junkie, serves her right
I saw her jagging up last night

Well let me put to rest your fears
I haven't used needles for many years
So why all the nasty lies?
Is that the way they get their highs?

I had great problems and that's no fiction
That was the cause of my addiction
Now I'm drug free an' trying hard
Even though my life's been marred

Oh, if you could only see
What your bad treatment's done to me
I hurt, I cry, I ache inside
I've even thought of suicide

But this is my life mate, it's my lot
No matter what disease I've got
I've got to keep going
I've got to keep trying

Even though the shit keeps flying
Why don't they look and see
There is no difference between them and me?
I ain't no dog, no snake, no louse
And no I'm not a little mouse

And if it's my disease your seeing
Look again I'm a HUMAN BEING

August 1989

Quick put the barricades
Here comes that thing with AIDS

That walking talking deadly germ
There's no way our respect she'll earn

Look out she might breathe on you
And you will be an outcast too

This is not fiction, this is fact
This is the way some people react

Fortunately some understand
They're not afraid to hold my hand

I pray one day there will be a cure
As my days are getting fewer

Not just for AIDS you understand
But for all the ignorance across the land

August 1989

I wish I could stop reverting
To feelings which are disconcerting
I don't want to backslide, I want to go on
I don't want to be anyone's pawn

Or be manipulated, worked like a puppet
If that's the offer, then you can stuff it
I want to be whole, I want to be real
And cope with these feelings that I feel

I don't want to go through life having to depend
On a liquid green bottle I thought was my friend
I thought it loved me and would never forsake me
But all it did was tear and rape me

I thought I was the one that was doing the using
I thought it was great I thought I was cruising
But my liquid green friend was telling me lies
She put a shield right over my eyes

I couldn't see my life was in bits
Or the things around me I was in the pits
Until one day there was nowhere to hide
I had to do something and swallow my pride

So I came to this rehab to get myself cleaned
And off the drug I was slowly weaned
Sometimes my mind it starts to pretend
That I need her back, my little green friend

But I don't need her, I see that myself
All she can do is ruin my health
I know I've got a lot of work still to do
But without friends like that I know I'll get through

At the moment I'm coping I'm happy and fine
But taking it slowly one day at a time
As each day goes by I'm feeling stronger
Soon I'll be her prisoner no longer

August 1989

Tell me Doc, will I die soon
I wish I knew I'd be over the moon
All the hurt, pain would be gone
Go on please tell me have I got long?

The heartache and sadness a thing of the past
Eternal sleep and peace at last
Can I have some AZT with the hope that the side effects
They would kill me

I can't get free from this depression
This fuckin' disease has become an obsession
I lie awake and think of AIDS
All sense of being rational quickly fades

In the morning I pray and hope
I try to be optimistic so I can cope
I put on a smile and say I'm alright
I try to forget my pain of the night

But it's not just my nights, it's also my days
When I'm constantly thinking about this AIDS
I want to scream and tear my hair out
What is this fuckin' existence about?

Trying to live is very hard
When I know this syndrome has marked my card
The rejection, the fear is making me ill
I feel like giving up, I'm losing my will

Should I take some drugs and try to forget
Unfortunately its something my budget won't let
Run to the City to get a script for Meth
At least I'll be calm for my encounter with Death

What should I do, ask for help
And in my face another skelp?
You're just weak, you can't cope
Thats what you get for taking Dope

You're just a junkie, it's what you deserve
Now you want help, what a nerve
Go away, don't make a fuss
We're busy people, don't bother us

We don't really care about your pain
Now go away and don't complain
I don't know just what to do
There must be an answer I wish I knew

I'm not living I feel I'm dying
I've no will left to keep on trying
My nerves are shattered my heart is broken
With all the bad words that have been spoken

At the moment I feel I need a crutch
'Cos this pain and confusion is all too much
The worth of my life is easy to measure
While I'm under all this fuckin' pressure

It's not even worth one millimetre
'Cos in has crept my defeator
I'm sitting here ripped up inside
And contemplating suicide

I'm sick of fighting and always losing
It's very hard and most confusing
Should I wait for death to come to me?
Will this disease set me free?

There is no more to be said on this issue
Except, Shit, Quick, pass me a tissue
The price of the battle has been a lot
It's taken everything I've got

August 1989

ARC and AIDS and HIV
This bloody thing is killing me

But can I ask this little question
Could it all be autosuggestion?

Is this diarrhoea for real
Or was it just that Indian meal?

I know I sneeze an awful lot
But is it this disease I've got?

I was on pills to put weight on
Or was that just another con?

They gave me placebos this I know
'Cos my consultant told me so

I'm not being diplomatic
I just want to know if it's psychosomatic

August 1989

Afterword – The Way Forward

The lack of clear data on the numbers and location of children and young people affected by HIV/AIDS (in particular the lack of figures for particular age groups) is a major barrier to effective planning. However, the relatively small number of children currently infected is a 'smoke screen' in the light of:

- probable under-reporting; and
- the much wider numbers of children directly affected by living in a household with another family member with HIV or AIDS.

In effect accurate data on children and HIV/AIDS *must* acknowledge the family context of prevention and management. It is unlikely that the health care and community care plans required under the NHS and Community Care Act will adequately reflect the needs of these families without clearer guidance on prevalence and geographical location of parents and children.

Many of the problems surrounding HIV/AIDS and children relate to the associated economic and social disadvantage related to chronic and terminal illness and disability. We need to learn quickly from the extensive data on the lives and needs of families with other disabilities or health problems so that we may develop comprehensive and flexible provision which acknowledges a wide range of cultural, personal and social life styles and which builds upon the strengths of families and the local community.

There is an immediate need for accessible, integrated, local and good quality services which are *child and family-centred*. The Children Act 1989 offers a legal and conceptual framework for supporting *children in need* within their families. The Children Act's emphasis on active partnerships with parents and the need to collaborate with education and health authorities should be seen as an opportunity to plan more coherent policies for the future and to ensure that provision for children and families reflects the best of current *child*-care policy and practice. The provision of day care, financial assistance, holiday provision, respite care, counselling and advice (amongst many other services) are all crucial to the effective management of children with HIV/AIDS. But this provision should not be seen as a 'separate service' which further isolates children and family and ignores the existing resources of, for example, family centres, playgroups and the Education Authority and District Health Authority.

All children's services contacted in our Survey identified a key principle of the Children Act, namely the need *to* listen to children. There is currently a major shortfall in counselling skills and professional training in this area.

Health education is crucial not only in prevention of HIV but also to enable children's services to work proactively with affected children and families. The education services offer major challenges and opportunities for supporting children with HIV – but frequently receive little age-appropriate and relevant advice on pastoral care and HIV in children and families.

Our report suggests that there are growing numbers of children and families who are socially isolated because of certain specific factors in addition to HIV/AIDS which inhibit them from gaining access to appropriate support and help. These families are likely to live in smaller communities and towns, rural areas or inner cities.

Many are distant from major treatment centres and may fear to reveal their HIV status because of anxiety about rejection and ostracism. Some families will come from the Black and minority ethnic communities, about which we have very little information. Black families may be even more reluctant to use services because of the risk of racism in their local communities or language difficulties.

Some children and young people affected by HIV will live with substitute (foster) families or in residential settings. There is an urgent need to plan services to support children and young people who have no natural family and who must therefore live away from home. Most of the current expertise with separated children with HIV is in the field of young children. There is therefore an urgent need to look at the special needs of adolescents and young people and to develop services which are age-appropriate and address both prevention and treatment.

There is currently no specific organisation to act as an advocate and source of information on *children's* issues relating to AIDS/HIV. The majority of influential AIDS/HIV groups focus upon adults and adult services. The report emphasises the urgent need for a resource and database on HIV and AIDS and children, which can meet the special needs of professionals, statutory services, voluntary organisations and consumers. There is a parallel need for a *Standing Conference* on children's services, to help shape and to contribute to the development of policy and practice in this area.

In conclusion, the report identifies a number of effective, consumer-sensitive and child and family focused services. We need to learn from the positive practices already in operation and to see HIV/AIDS as an integral part of all provision for children and families.

We must also acknowledge that Paediatric AIDS and the management of AIDS/HIV in *children* is different in many respects to that of adults. The legal, ethical, practical and emotional issues around HIV/AIDS and children require a radical reassessment. This report should be seen as the start of a major agenda for change.

Philippa Russell,
Director, Voluntary Council
for Handicapped Children

Appendix 1   Sample questionnaire

National Children's Bureau Information Sheet – HIV Infection and Children

> This sheet has been completed by:
>
> Name:
>
> Organisation:
>
> Address:
>
> Tel:

1 Approximately how many children and/or young people are you currently providing services for in relation to HIV/AIDS?

2 What is the age range?   0–1 yr
                                  1–5 yrs
                                  5–11 yrs
                                  11–18 yrs

3 What services do you provide? Including work with parents, carers, families.

4 In your experience what specific needs do they have? (Please tick)

    Medical/health care monitoring

    Nursing

    Social care – residential, day care, foster care,
        family support, adoption

    Respite care

    Educational

    Housing

    Legal advice

    Welfare benefits

Employment

Social work support

Counselling

5 List any other needs not already mentioned above.

6 Are there any special issues which pose problems for the agency in relation to HIV concerns?

   (*If yes*, can you say what they are)

7 Has your agency developed any written policy guidelines on HIV, or published any pamphlets, information etc?

   (*If yes*, can you describe what aspects are covered, and for whom are they intended, eg. staff
   children
   parents, families, carers

8 Has your agency developed any specific initiatives, projects or services including joint work with other agencies etc?

   (*If yes*, – could you say briefly what these developments are.)

9 Are you satisfied with the current level of services provided by your agency or are there specific initiatives you would like to develop?

10 Are there other needs which your agency cannot meet but which you feel should be developed in the future?

   (*If yes*, would you like to say what these are?)

11 What financial resources are available for the development of work in relation to HIV services?

12 Finally, are there any other concerns or comments which you would like to mention?

Appendix 2   Questionnaire analysis

This appendix contains a brief summary of the main findings which emerged from the responses of the National Children's Bureau members who replied to the questionnaire. The analysis has been grouped according to issues rather than to specific question numbers (see Appendix 1 for sample questionnaire).

Number of returned completed questionnaires

Breakdown by agency	Numbers	%
Health authorities	59	40.4
Social service department	33	22.6
Voluntary organisations	31	21.2
Education authorities	14	9.5
Others	9	6.1
Total	146	

Comment

Forty per cent of all replies came from medical staff in health care settings and 43 per cent were from voluntary and social services. Only nine per cent of local education authorities reponded, although they are the most likely after District Health Authorities to have direct involvement with children and young people with HIV, as the majority of children with HIV are in the school population. The cumulative total number of infected children aged 14 years or less with haemophilia and HIV for the UK as of 30 September 1990 was 407. The total numer of AIDS cases were 49.[2]

Number of agencies providing direct care to children in relation to HIV (Q1)

Thirty-six agencies are presently giving a direct service to children with HIV, representing 24.6 per cent of all respondents.

Breakdown by agency	%
Health services	65.8
Voluntary and social services	28.5
Others	5.7
Number of children	
Number of children known to have HIV	123
Number of children alleged to have HIV (but not verifiable)	80
Total	203

Comment

It was surprising that nearly a quarter of agencies responding are already having some direct experience of working with children with HIV infection. It is also possible that some of these children are being seen by different agencies and therefore appearing more than once in agencies' statistics. Many agencies have a policy of confidentiality and non-disclosure of HIV status but nevertheless indicated that, although unable to verify the HIV status of individuals, issues relating to HIV were often of considerable concern to young poeple and those who worked with them. This concern was, in some cases, having a major impact on agency developments.

Age range of children seen (Q2)

Age range of children seen	Number	%
0–1 years	15	7.3
0–5 years	48	23.6
5–11 years	21	10.3
11–18 years	119	59.0

Comment

Despite the difficulty of attaching too much reliance on the actual number of children with HIV in the 11–18-year-old group, the response does mirror the approximate distribution of HIV infection in children and young people according to the CDSC returns for the end of September 1989.

Range of services provided (Q3)

Comment

The range of services provided included:

- direct care and work with children and young people in health, education and personal social services in residential and day care and field settings;
- support services for families, fostering and adoption, childcare minders;
- health education, promotion and training;
- coordinating and planning services;
- specialist services for one client group, for example, drug rehabilitation, offenders, out-reach and community work with young people or the young homeless;
- welfare benefits advice;
- educational research.

Meeting service needs (Q4)

Comment

The majority of agencies felt that they were currently providing a reasonable level of services in line with agency functions and known need. The exceptions were the smaller voluntary agencies providing out-reach work, or working with street-based agencies, drop-in centres and crisis centres for the homeless or runaway teenagers. They were aware that they were not able to meet the immediate needs of vulnerable young people for housing, shelter and protection, and felt under great pressure to respond to crises without adequate staffing and resources.

Some agencies did express apprehension about their preparedness for work with HIV clients and their families. They felt unsure about the level of services provided, and whether they would be adequate if there was an increase in HIV work.

Most respondents ticked all areas of need mentioned in question four but articulated the following needs most frequently. The need:

- to develop planned integrated childcare policies and services;
- to provide flexible day care – such as drop-in centres – especially for family support and local groups, including improved:
  - childcare facilities;
  - support for carers;
  - support for young drug misusers;
  - peer group support;
  - provision for the young homeless;
- for provision of hospice care and respite care for parents and children with HIV;
- to improve housing provision for the young homeless and vulnerable young people such as those leaving care;
- for provision of holidays for children and families;
- to develop and integrate sex education within schools as part of the core curriculum;
- for learning and developing skills in communicating with young children and adolescents;

- for time to counsel children about HIV concerns;
- to develop bereavement counselling services for children, as well as parents;
- for time to offer and receive spiritual support.

Particular needs, issues and concerns (Q5, 6 and 10)

Respondents were asked to identify particular areas of needs and concerns and to speculate about forward planning. Those most frequently mentioned related to:

- Children:
  - developing counselling and communication skills;
  - counselling on illness, bereavement, care and treatment, sex and sexuality, health education, and drug misuse;
  - working with abused children, or those with special needs or children with behavioural problems;
  - relationships with school services;
  - communicating with families of children with HIV;
  - legal rights of children, particularly relating to treatment and informed consent.
- Families:
  Need to develop a more family-centred service for support of child and family networks. Particularly in relationship to drug misusing families.
- Drug misuse:
  Many staff expressed a lack of confidence and skills in working with drug misusers, and their families. Knowledge, information and resources on drug misuse should be expanded.
  It was acknowledged that services for drug misusers were inadequate, and that these should be expanded to meet the needs of users. It was also generally agreed that they should be informal, non-judgemental and accessible.
- Training:
  Staff development and training was considered very important in preparing staff to work confidently in HIV related services. Most people felt that training opportunities were too often limited to 'awareness' days. There was a need to develop on-going training to take account of changing needs, new information and constant staff turnover. Concern was expressed by small voluntary organisations who lacked financial resources to mount adequate training programmes.
- Confidentiality:
  Most agencies continued to feel worried about all issues concerned with confidentiality – including:
  - storing and recording confidential information systems;
  - the developing and implementing of 'confidentiality' policies and guidance;
  - how best to resolve professional dilemmas about 'who needs to know?';
  - rights of children, parents and foster parents and adopters;
  - recognising the tensions and conflicts in controlling and containing confidential information, and concern about unforeseen care issues for children, including monitoring changes in health and protecting them from avoidable risks.

- Housing:
  Concerns were uppermost for the needs of homeless young people and
  absconders or runaway children for adequate housing provision, shelter and
  support organisations offering crisis care.

Agency policies on HIV (including information materials) (Q7)

Agency policies on HIV (including information materials)	%
Agencies with written policies for staff	68
Agencies with written policies for children's needs	6.5
Agencies with written policies for carers	16.2
Agencies with written policies for parents	7.3
No reply on policies	2

Comment

It was surprising and disturbing that only 6.5 per cent of agencies had developed any
material which was directly targeted on providing information for children
themselves. Where material had been produced it tended to be health education for
young people on safer sex and safer drug use, or information for boys with
haemophilia. Few agencies saw children as a 'needy' group except as 'receptors' for
health education messages. They were more likely to be seen as 'transmitters' of
HIV than people with feelings, views and needs of their own.

Approximately two thirds of all agencies, identified staff group needs as a priority
area. This reflects the need to develop 'HIV Awareness Training' in order to combat
myths, fears and prejudice about working with HIV anti-body positive clients.
Policies mainly covered areas of health, safety and infection control; confidentiality
and testing; training strategies; non-discriminatory practices and equal opportunities. Particular policies for children in care including guidelines on fostering and
adoption, testing and confidentiality had been developed in *some* local authority
social service departments.

Policies on confidentiality and testing were not always so well defined in health
services or education settings, and it was less clear from the replies whether staff
received guidance on these matters.

In many agencies health education and prevention policies were initiated by
health promotion units in health authorities, in some localities social services took
the lead.

Voluntary organisations were more likely to have produced 'user friendly'
material for staff and carers, and to place greater emphasis on sex education and
preventative health policies and on staff training for all workers.

Education authorities were more likely to have emphasised health safety and
infection control procedures and policies on sex education for teachers, parents and
governors.

Developing initiatives (Q8)

Comments

Many organisations provided detailed information on specific projects or joint work with other agencies. These included:

- theatre in education on HIV in schools, youth clubs and community centres;
- publishing educational materials, newsletters and 'comics'; and making tapes and videos;
- out-reach work with drug misusers, including needle exchange, condom distribution and work with young male and female prostitutes. Developing training initiatives across health and social services;
- much of this work appeared to be exciting and innovative, particularly in the area of health education campaigns. However, there was a paucity of evidence on monitoring and assessing the effectiveness of these approaches.

Inter-agency strategic planning: Coordination and liaison

Three distinct models of inter-agency planning and coordination of policies and services were identified by the survey. These were:

- The Strathclyde Model – Towards An Inter-Agency Strategy in Strathclyde – [61] promotes a multi-agency and multi-faceted approach. It is predominantly led by the Health and Social Work Boards, but invites participation from voluntary organisations such as Scottish AIDS Monitor, Helplines and the Church;
- The Manchester Aids In Education Group[62] – brings together education services, health promotion units and health services, with an emphasis on health education for young people in school and the community;
- The National Council for Childcare Voluntary Organisations – brings together voluntary organisations in childcare around a 'special interest' group to promote information and exchange and training and practice development of services for their own organisations.

The first two models, although they promote inter-agency approaches and 'invite' voluntary organisations to be involved in planning, are predominantly focusing on the interests of the lead agencies and voluntary organisations are not seen as equal partners.

In the third model the special interest group is concerned with developing consistent policies and detailed guidance on HIV to all its members for one client group, that is young children. These models, together with other models, need to be assessed for their effectiveness in developing the best services for children.

Interestingly, no model was presented that brought together health, education and the personal social services in one planning arena.

Developing services (Q9)

It was suggested that the following developments were needed:

- an HIV Paediatric Information Forum – to disseminate, coordinate and up-date research and information and initiatives on the medical and social care and treatment of children;

- published guidance on best childcare policies and practice. This should include legal rights of children on testing and confidentiality which can be applied in all health, education and social services settings;
- strategic planning for integrating Child Health Services within the reorganised NHS structure;
- flexible day care provision which is family-centred – including respite care, crèche facilities, nurseries, sheltered housing and drop-in centres. Drug misusing families needed family support resources that were friendly and non-judgemental. Fears that children may be taken into care prevented many families seeking help from social services;
- mobile out-reach resources for young people, including transport such as minibuses, health care teams working with 'runaways' and vulnerable young people associating with prostitution and drug misuse. Training facilities for developing social and life skills for rehabilitation of young people;
- provision of appropriate community-based services for minority ethnic communities, including increasing the number of Black staff, specialist link workers and advocates, and translation services;
- training programmes for all staff who work directly with children on communication skills, including counselling children with long-term illness and disabilities, bereavement, sexual counselling, social skills training and drug misuse;
- practice skills on work with children with severe behaviour problems;
- improved services and training for children with special needs;
- update staff training regularly – particularly in drug misuse, HIV care and treatment, and work with young people and with minority ethnic groups – taking account of high staff turn-over and burn-out;
- monitoring childcare practice and standards in the private sector including concerns about training staff and implementing effective HIV policies.

Developing services and special concerns (Qs 10 and 12)

Comments

There was considerable consensus on areas that need to be developed, falling into the two major categories of concerns and developing services.

Concerns

The most commonly expressed concerns related to combating discrimination, stigmatisation and prejudice. Concern was also expressed about:

- keeping up-to-date with HIV information and research;
- staff stress and burn-out;
- meeting the needs of special groups of children, such as absconding young people who are homeless and vulnerable, and may be less likely to protect themselves from HIV transmission, because of risk activities such as prostitution and drug misuse. Similar fears were expressed for young people who may have experienced violent and abusing sexual behaviour from adults.

Lack of understanding and knowledge about HIV policies in schools, and criticism of the role of school doctors, nurses and teachers in relating to children and parents with HIV were areas of concern mentioned by respondents.

Concern was also expressed about some minority ethnic families who may be particularly isolated as the result of their HIV status, and unable to seek support from families or obtain counselling from trained Black staff. Fear that HIV is becoming over-medicalised would seem to be widely felt.

Resources available for HIV services (Q11)

Comment

When asked to comment on the level of funds available for HIV services, there was a marked difference in levels of satisfaction from agency to agency. In general, health authorities felt well resourced and some even felt over-endowed for the work being undertaken. However, in districts with a high HIV profile of work, there was concern at the reluctance on the part of some managers to recognise and resource staff giving direct care and counselling to clients. These staff often felt over-stretched and unable to cope with demands for information, advice and guidance.

Voluntary organisations most often complained about lack of resources and felt unable to meet the work-load demands for expanded provision. These organisations are most likely to be small organisations working directly with vulnerable groups, such as out-reach work with young people or specialist groups like haemophilia sufferers.

There would appear to be an urgent need to acknowledge the intensity of this work and provide more resources for trained staff. Information services are also needed. It is also necessary to recognise that different services should be developed to meet different needs – such as drop-in centres and mobile primary health care teams for the young homeless or drug misusers.

Conclusions

The questionnaire illuminated a wide spectrum of agency practices, policies and needs. Many of the issues raised represented similar concerns to those identified in specific areas of the main study and do seem to mirror experiences elsewhere.

Perhaps the most worrying finding of the questionnaire was the lack of any clear, coherent policies for direct work with children. Very few agencies seemed to have the skills or confidence to involve children actively as participants in areas of decision-making, treatment or care plans. Children were least likely to be consulted or their views and opinions sought. It was as if they were invisible.

There is a dearth of suitable information and material for primary school children. Communicating with children and developing a child-centred approach is given a low priority in most agencies.

Staff fears and anxieties dominate and reflect many of the uncertainties and the de-skilling process that has followed the advent of HIV and AIDS.

The survey prompted respondents to comment on key areas. The following section identifies these concerns under specific topic headings.

Issues and comments

Policies

- Paediatric guidelines – especially on clinical aspects of HIV and treatment needed for children in care.
- Relating to and treating drug users – most staff feel uneasy and lack confidence and skills. Agency policies need to address this need.
- Better coordination between services – agencies are unaware of internal policies.
- HIV testing is still an uncertain area – the issues surrounding children for adoption/fostering, for example. Sometimes the issues are concerning the HIV status of foster parents or adopters.
- Some Health and Safety guidelines on staff/child protection are difficult to implement – for example, an adventure playground setting.
- HIV issues should be integrated into all aspects of training, and all policies on non-discrimination, equal opportunities, preventative health care.
- Professional isolation – within agencies and between agencies – hinders the development of good services.
- Poverty and social deprivation are still major concerns which policies for HIV have to address.

Resources

- Emergency funds needed to coordinate and centralise funding and avoid piecemeal negotiations and time-wasting procedures.
- Voluntary organisations are under funded, despite giving a great deal of direct care – they often carry an excessive burden of responsibilities that is not formally recognised.
- More resources needed for childminders.
- Developing more day care, drop-in centres for vulnerable families.
- Need to provide more out-reach services – counselling on safer sex, condom provision, and needle exchanges – requires adequate resourcing. Need for mobile services for young people – such as primary health care.

Children

- Need to develop material for children with learning difficulties and special needs.
- Counselling for bereaved children should be provided in all agencies involved with children.
- Communicating with children
  – 'how to tell' children with HIV;
  – giving career advice for children in care;
  – legal rights of children in relation to testing, consent to treatment and so on;
  – role of the Courts in counselling on sex/sexuality.
- Hospice care for children with AIDS is needed.
- Working with abused children, the young homeless, children at risk, and children in care. Some children have no social worker – education staff shortages.
- Developing specific services for children – in DHAs – child health strategies – appear to be lacking. There is little evidence of planning mechanisms and policies.

- How to protect and supervise children in private placements – especially handicapped children and children with special needs.
- Children with haemophilia, and their special needs in schools and the community. Health education needs are not always being met.
- Need for clearer guidelines on good childcare practice, including legal rights – for example, acknowledging differences in legal status of a minor in Scotland and England and Wales and Northern Ireland.
- Female/male prostitution in young people. There is concern about their health education – safer sex. They are less likely, as a group, to protect themselves – because of their lifestyle.

Families

- Developing guidance and information for families and creating support mechanisms.
- Working with families with HIV – parents and/or children – developing support services.

Education

- Confidentiality – better record keeping required. Who needs to know? – concerns about school staff.
- Educating school staff about HIV in-service policies, including dentists and nurses.
- All agencies need to develop better links with schools and education services in relation to HIV issues.
- The role of the school nurse needs to be clarified in relation to HIV policies. Many schools do not have school nurses, so how will the health of school children be monitored?
- The School Health Services should ensure that all school dentists have received adquate training and briefing on HIV policies, including in relation to children with special needs

Health education

- Improved health education and more funding for LEAs needed. Health education should be a *core* subject in every school curriculum.
- Need to develop more research into teenage sexuality.
- Health Education Programmes. These could be more imaginative – such as Theatre projects; the Inner Circle (Barnet); held in informal settings in youth clubs and so on; peer group education; newsletters; and so on. Must develop a sex education framework for prevention of transmission – it is not enough just to concentrate on HIV issues.

Drug misuse

- In working with drug misusers, there is a need for residential units for parents and children. Drug services – 50 per cent of users have children, so their needs must be addressed. Also more support is needed for ex-users, and for family units.

Minority ethnic groups

- Problems about refugee status, and immigration laws are even more crucial when a child is HIV positive. The fear of repatriation is real and can equate with no treatment.
- Developing better health education programmes for minority ethnic community members – concern about how to reach drug misusers from different cultures, and provide accessible information in other languages.

Housing

- Housing is a major issue for young vulnerable people such as drug misusers, teenage run-aways, and the homeless.

Training

- Developing more information and training for staff – including addressing the training needs of carers and volunteers.

Appendix 3   HIV statistics – a different perspective

North West Thames HIV Prevention Letter, Winter 1989/90. Issue 1

HIV statistics – a different perspective

In this edition we present the UK antibody positive test reports collected by the Communicable Diseases Surveillance Centre (CDSC) and the Communicable Diseases (Scotland) Unit up to the quarter ending 30 September 1989. The data is presented both in the standard table used by the CDSC and in a new format devised by Clive Stevens, Senior Programme Officer with the HEA AIDS division.

- The key aspect of the Stevens model is that it attempts to make a clear distinction between "probable route of infection" and whether a person labels themselves as gay, bisexual, injecting drug user or heterosexual. This is designed both to emphasise the idea of "high risk behaviour", challenging the notion of "high risk groups", and to encourage people to recognise that the way a person becomes infected with HIV does not necessarily determine the route of transmission to others, (eg. an injecting drug user could become infected through using contaminated works and then pass on the infection to a sexual partner). This has implications for prevention message.
- CDSC stats are cumulated including deaths. This leads to a false picture of the present situation. The Stevens model shows only people living, to indicate more closely the nature of the epidemic now.
- The CDSC table sometimes excludes Scotland. Stevens points out that this division is not appropriate in "national" data, in his model Scotland is always included.
- Stevens also argues that it is illogical to combine data on gay and bisexual men. Ideally his table would separate these two groups. Similarly he points out that the current data doees not indicate how many gay or bisexual men become infected via blood products or how many children with haemophilia are included in the heterosexual "Factor 8" category of the CDSC table.
- To provide this data the CDSC would have to make major alterations to their HIV and AIDS data gathering systems.

HIV antibody positive persons reported by patient characteristics for the UK: cumulative totals up to the end of September 1989*

Transmission Category	Male	Female	Unknown	Total
Homo/Bisexual	5390	0	0	5390
Intravenous drug abuser (IVDA)	1106	541	31	1678
Homo/bisexual and IVDA	93	0	0	93
Haemophiliac**	1088	7	1	1096
Recipient of blood	60	48	2	110
Heterosexual contact:				
Partner(s) with above	14	119	1	134
risk factors;				
Others:				
Possibly infected abroad;	216	127	7	350
No evidence of exposure abroad;	18	13	2	33
Undetermined	93	104	0	197
Child of at risk/infected parent	49	54	33	136
Multiple risks	7	0	0	7
Other/undetermined	1668	188	138	1994
Total	9802	1201	215	11218

* For the first time, reports from Scotland are included in this table.
** The actual number of known HIV infected haemophiliacs is greater. A number of persons in the undetermined exposure category are thought to be haemophiliacs who were tested in 1985.

Human Immunodeficiency Virus (HIV) Antibody Reports for United Kingdom
(*Cumulative figures, excludes deaths up to September 30 1989*)

Probable infection route	Heterosexual Male	Heterosexual Female	Heterosexual Gender not known	Bisexual Homosexual Male	Bisexual Homosexual Female	Child Boy	Child Girl	Child Gender not known	Other/ insufficient information collected	Gender Totals Male	Gender Totals Female	Gender Totals Gender not known	Totals
Sexual	303	340	10	4282	–	–	–	–		4585	340	10	4935
Sharing injecting drug use equipment	1085	530	31	76	–	–	–	–		1161	530	31	1722
Blood/Blood products — Blood Components	42	34	2	(?)	(?)	–	–	–		42	34	2	78
Blood/Blood products — Factor 8 + 9 (Previously infected)	987	6	1	(?)	(?)					987	6	1	993 (1072)
Child at risk from infected mother						46	46	33		46	46	33	125
Multiple risks									7	7			7
Other/Insufficient information collected									1969	1645	186	138	1969
Gender totals	2417	910	44	4358	–	46	46	33	1976	8473	1142	215	
Totals	3371			4358			125		1976				9830

Full details of Clive Stevens' work on data collection and presentation are contained in his paper '*The Presentation of HIV/AIDS statistics – a re-examination*'. N.B. From January 1991 The PHLS CDSC and CD (Scotland) U will present the statistics for HIV/AIDS in a revised format (*see* Appendix 4).

Appendix 4   New AIDS figures

The words homosexual, bisexual, and hetrosexual are missing from a new table giving the total number of AIDS cases reported up to the end of last month. In their place are the exposure categories of "Sexual intercourse between men" and "Sexual intercourse between men and women"; it is argued that this "emphasises more directly how persons probably acquired the virus."

Altogether 1276 new cases of AIDS were reported in the United Kingdom in 1990, a 51% increase over the number of new cases reported in 1988 (itself up 12% on

Cases of AIDS in the United Kingdom by probable route of HIV infection (cumulative totals up to end of December 1990)

	Men (n=3895)	Women (n=203)	Total (n=4098)	Deaths (n=2256)
Sexual intercourse				
Between men	3234		3234	1789
Between men and women*				
"High risk" partner†	11	23	34	19
Other partner abroad	145	63	208	93
Other partner UK	13	13	26	9
Injecting drug use (IDU)	123	38	161	70
IDU and sexual intercourse between men	61		61	32
Blood				
Blood factor (eg haemophiliacs)	225	3	228	156
Blood or tissue transfer (eg transfusion)				
Abroad	13	24	37	23
UK	16	14	30	22
Mother to child	15	21	36	15
Other or undetermined	39	4	43	28

*Includes men and women who had sexual intercourse with injecting drug users or with those infected by contaminated blood and women who had intercourse with bisexual men.
†Includes people without other identified risks from, or who have lived in, countries where the main route of HIV-1 transmission is through sexual intercourse between men and women.

1987). Exposure categories experienced different rates of increase between 1989 and 1990: a rise of 44% for sexual intercourse between men and women, and 102% for injecting drug use.

The designations "homosexual men" and the rest reappear in a new table in the report listing cases of AIDS in adults by sexual orientation. The table was compiled to show the potential for further transmission of HIV-1 in the United Kingdom through hetrosexual intercourse. It shows that 271 (22%) of the new AIDS cases in 1990 were reported in hetrosexual men and women. This category includes those infected through injecting drugs or by contaminated blood.

The number and proportion of new cases of AIDS actually acquired by hetrosexual intercourse (and reported in 1990) was much smaller (123, 10%). Most of these cases were infected with HIV by partners living abroad (see figure).

– TONY DELAMOTHE

AIDS acquired by heterosexual contact, new cases by quarter

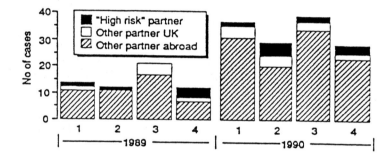

AIDS acquired by homosexual contact, new cases by quarter

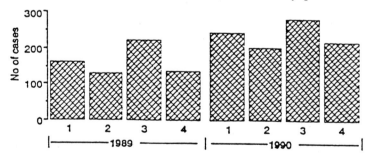

Prepared from voluntary confidential reports by clinicians and microbiologists sent directly to the PHLS Communicable Disease Surveillance Centre (081 200-6868) and the Communicable Diseases (Scotland) Unit (041 946-7120) and from monthly returns by paediatricians to the British Paediatric Surveillance Unit (071 935-1866).

References

(1) Day, N.E. (Chairman), *Acquired Immune Deficiency Syndrome in England And Wales To End 1991.* Report of Working Group Convened by Director of Public Health Laboratory Service. PHLS Communicate Disease Surveillance Centre: 1990.

(2) *AIDS/HIV Quarterly Surveillance Tables, The Data To End September 1990.* Public Health Laboratory Service AIDS Centre and the Communicative Diseases (Scotland) Unit: 9: 1990.

(3) Department of Health and Welsh Office, *Short-term prediction of HIV Infection and AIDS in England and Wales.* HMSO: 1988.

(4) Parkside Health Authority, *AIDSPLAN: A Planning Model for HIV/AIDS Services for Parkside Health Authority.* Project Report: October 1989 (Unpublished).

Riverside Health Authority, *HIV and AIDS, A Strategy For Care 1989-1994.* (Unpublished)

(5) House of Commons Social Services Committee. *Third Report: Problems Associated with AIDS:* II. HMSO: 1987.

(6) See reference (2).

(7) House of Commons Social Services Committee. *Seventh Report: AIDS.* HMSO: 1989.

(8) Peckham, C.S. and others, Prevalence of Maternal HIV infection based on unlinked anonymous testing of newborn babies. *Lancet* no 8688 pp 516-19: 3 March 1990.

(9) Davison, C.F. and others, HIV Infection in Pregnant Women and Children in the UK and Irish Republic. *Archives of AIDS Research*, 4 p 199: 1990.

(10) PHLS AIDS Centre at the Communicable Diseases Surveillance Centre and Communicable Disease (Scotland) Unit. *Format of regular tables summarising data on reported AIDS cases and HIV-1 antibody positive persons.* CDR 1, Review Number 1.

(11) Stevens, C., The Prevention of HIV/AIDS Statistics. A Reexamination *North West Thames HIV Prevention Letter.* Winter 1989/90.

(12) *AIDS and Children. A Family Disease.* Panos Institute: 1989.

(13) European Collaborative Study. Children Born to Women with HIV-1 Infection: Natural History and Risk of Transmission. *Lancet* no 8736, pp 253-60: Feb 1991.

(14) Stevens, A. and others, HIV Testing in Ante-natal Clinics: the Impact on Women. *AIDS Care,* 1, 2, pp 165-71: 1989.

(15) Johnstone, D. and others, Women's Knowledge of their HIV Antibody State: It's Effect on their Decision Whether to Continue Pregnancy. *BMJ* 6716, pp 23-4: 6 Jan 1990.

(16) Johnstone, F.D. and others, Does Infection with HIV Affect the Outcome of Pregnancy? *BMJ,* p 296, p 467: 13 Feb 1988.

(17) Sherr, L., *AIDS and HIV Infection In Mothers And Babies:* Blackwell: 1991.

(18) Mok, J. and others, *The Management Of Children Born To Human Immunodeficiency Virus Seropositive Women.* Conference at Queen Charlotte's Hospital.

(19) Jones, F. and others, Unintended Pregnancy. Contraceptive Practice and Family Planning Services in Developed Countries *in Family Planning Perspectives,* 20, 2: Alan Guttmacher Institute March/April 1988.

(20) Kenmir, B., Family Planning Clinic Cuts. Family Planning Association. *Times:* 5 June 1990.

(21) Bird, G., Immunologist Lecture at Edinburgh University Conference. *Times:* 5 June 1990.

(22) OPCS, *The Prevalence of Disability Among Children.* HMSO Report No 3: 1989.

OPCS, *The Financial Circumstances Of Families With Disabled Children Living In Private Households*. HMSO Report No 5: 1989.

OPCS, *Disabled Children: Services, Transport and Education*. HMSO Report No 6: 1989.

(23) AIDS Group of the UK Haemophilia Centre Directors with the Cooperation of the United Haemophilia Centre Directors. *Prevalence of antibody and HIV in Haemophiliacs in the United Kingdom: a second survey*. Clinical Lab. Haematology 1988, 10, pp 187-191.

(24) *Socio-Economic Background of People with Haemophilia and HIV in Comparison to the Estimated Population of 15-year-old+ males*. Haemophiliacs Society: 1988.

(25) Richards, J., and Nitabach, L., AIDS: Be Prepared. *Care Weekly* no 53 p 10: 21 Oct 1988.

(26) Newman, C., *Young Runaways*. Children's Society: 1989.

(27) Kinnell, H., *Risky Business: Prostitutes, Clients and HIV in Birmingham*. Central Birmingham Health Authority.

(28) Hayes, C., and Wright, A., Preparations for Change in North West Hertfordshire *in Responding to the AIDS Challenge*. Health Education Authority/Longman: 1989.

(29) Regional Health Authorities on *AIDS (Control) Act* Report for 1 April 1988: 31 March 1989.

(30) Department of Health, *Support Grant for Social Services For People with AIDS and Related Expenditure: Financial Year 1989/90*. LAC (89)1: 1989.

(31) *Education (No 2) Act 1986*. Section 18: HMSO: 1986.

(32) See reference (8)

(33) Rogers, F., Paediatric HIV Infection: Epidiomilogy, Etiopathogenesis and Transmission *in Pediatric Annals*, 17, 5: 1988.

(34) Boland, M. G., and others, Children with HIV Infection: Collaborative Responsibilities of the Child Welfare and Medical Communities. *Social Work*, 33, 6, pp 504-9: 1988.

(35) Allen, D.A., and Green, V.P., Helping Children Cope with Stress. *Early Child Development and Care*, 37, pp1-11: 1988.

(36) Ward-Wimmer, D., Care of Children with HIV Infection. *Nursery Clinics of North America*, 23, 4: 1988.

(37) ILEA Health Education and Personal Development Advisory Team. *Sex Wise. A discussion document about sex education.* 1988.

(38) Boland, M.G., and others, Helping Children with AIDS: The Role of Child Welfare Worker. *Public Welfare.* Winter, 1987.

Kubler Ross, E., *On Children and Death.* Collier Books: 1983.

Judd, D. *Give Sorrow Words.* Face Association Books: 1989.

(39) See reference (38).

(40) Scottish Preschool Playgroups Association. A Play Group's Story. *Roundabout*, p8: May/June 1988.

(41) Aggleton, P. and others. *Your Choice for Life: An Evaluation of Responses to a Government Initiative on HIV/AIDS Education.* Goldsmiths College, University of London: 1989.

(42) DHSS Community Child Health Project (Riverside Area) *Coordinating Health Provision: Is it Child's Play?* October 1987.

(43) Hogg C. and Rodin, J., *Setting Standards for Children in Health Care.* National Association for the Welfare of Children in Hospital: 1990.

(44) Bloomsbury Parkside and Riverside Community Health Council, *HIV News*, 7, March 1990.

(45) Gibb, D., Manifestations and Management of HIV Infection of Children. *AIDS Letter*, 1990, 18, pp 1-3.

(46) Thornes, R. The care of dying children and their families, *Guidelines from British Paediatric Association.* King Edwards Hospital Fund for London, National Association of Health Authorities: NAHA: 1988.

(47) See reference (37).

(48) London Borough of Hammersmith and Fulham. Social Services Department, *Policy for the Provision of Services to HIV Positive Children, Young People and their Families.* 1988.

Lothian Regional Council. Social Work Department. *Children and Families HIV and AIDS.* Strathclyde Regional Council: 1989.

(49) See reference (48).

(50) Honigsbaum, N., *Living and Working with HIV. Training Guidance for Staff in the Personal Social Services*. Central Council for Education and Training in Social Work: 1989.

(51) *Children Act 1989*. HMSO: 1989.

(52) Hall, D. (ed), *Health for All Children: A Programme of Child Health Surveillance*. Oxford Medical Publications: 1989.

(53) Woodroffe, C., and Kurtz, Z., *Working for Children? Children's Services and the NHS Review*. Children's Policy Review Group, National Children's Bureau: 1989.

(54) Smith, R., *Impact of HIV on Pregnancy*. Lecture at conference on Pregnancy and HIV at St Mary's Hospital, London: 1 Feb 1990.

(55) Batty, D., *The Implications of AIDS for Children in Care*. British Agencies for Adoption and Fostering: 1987.

(56) General Medical Council. *HIV Infection and AIDS: The Ethical Considerations*. 1988

(57) Department of Education and Science, *A Health Education From 5 to 16* (Curriculum Matters 6). HMSO: 1986.

(58) See reference note (28).

(59) Septimus, A., Psycho-Social Aspects of Caring for Families of Infants with Human Immunodeficiency Virus. *Seminars in Perinatology*, 13, no.1, 1989. (Albert Einstein College of Medicine, Yeshiva University, Bronx N.Y.).

(60) US Department of Health and Human Services. Public Health Service. *Report of the Surgeon General's Workshop on Children with HIV Infection and their Families*. 6-9 April 1987.

(61) Strathclyde Regional Council. *HIV Infection and AIDS. Towards an Inter-Agency Strategy in Strathclyde*, November 1988.

(62) Manchester AIDS in Education Group. City of Manchester Education Committee. Education Offices. Crown Square, Manchester, M60 3BB.

Useful Organisations and Addresses

This list gives only a small selection of the national and local voluntary organisations in the field of AIDS/HIV and of children's services which can give help or advice. The majority can provide contacts in a statutory, professional or voluntary services and provide a wide range of information and printed material on current policy and practice in this area.

Aberlour Child Care Trust
Aberlour Child Care, 36 Park Terrace, Stirling, Scotland. Tel: 0786 50335.

AIDS Ahead
144 London Road, Northwich, Cheshire CW9 5HH.
Tel: 0606 47047.

AVERT
AIDS Education and Research Trust, PO Box 91,
Horsham RH13 7YR. Tel: 0403 864010.

Barnardo's
Barnardo's, Tanners Lane, Barkingside, Essex. Tel: 081 550 8822.

Black HIV/AIDS Network (BHAN)
111 Devonport Road, London W12 8PB.
Tel: 081-749 2828, 081-742 9223 (Helpline).

Blackliners
Brixton Enterprise Centre
444 Brixton Road, London SW9 8EJ.
Tel: 071-274 4000 Ex 217.

Body Positive
Body Positive, 51b Philbeach Gardens, London SW5 9EB. Tel:
Administration 071-835 1045, Helpline 071-373 9124 (run by and for
people who are HIV positive) Daily 7-10pm.

British Agencies for Adoption & Fostering (BAAF)
11 Southwark Street, London SE1 1RQ. Tel: 071-407 8800.

Cardiff AIDS Helpline
PO Box 348, Cardiff CF1 4XL.
Tel: 0222 223443.

Child Care
National Council of Voluntary Child Care Organisations, 8 Wakley
Street, London EC1V 7QE. Tel: 071-833 3319.

Children's Legal Centre
20 Compton Terrace, London N1.
Tel: 071-359 6251.

Family Planning Association Education Unit
27-35 Mortimer Street, London W1N 7RJ. Tel: 071-631 0555.

The Haemophilia Society
123 Westminster Bridge Road, London SE1 7HR.
Tel: 071-928 2020.

Health Education Authority
Hamilton House, Mabledon Place, London WC1.
Tel: 071-383 3833.

Immunity
Society for HIV Research and Education, BM Immunity,
London WC1N 3XX. Tel: 071-582 8829.

London Lesbian and Gay Switchboard
BM Switchboard, London WC1N 3XX. Tel: 071-837 7324.

London Lighthouse
111-117 Lancaster Road, London W11 1QT. Tel: 071-792 1200.

Mainliners
Unit 111, Enterprise Centre, 444 Brixton Road,
London SW9 8EJ. Tel: 071-274 4000 Ex 315.

Mildmay Mission Hospital
Hackney Road, London E2 7NA. Tel: 071-739 2331.

National AIDS Counselling Training Units
National AIDS Training Unit, St Charles' Hospital, Exmoor Street,
London W10 6DZ. Tel: 081-968 8514/5.

Boston General Hospital, Farnworth, Bolton BL4 0JR. Tel: 0204
390988.

National AIDS Helpline
Helpline: 0800 567 123, Free and confidential 24-hour telephone
advice for anyone who has questions or is worried about HIV/AIDS.
Cantonese Line: 0800 282 446, Tuesdays 6-10pm
Asian Line: 0800 282 445 (for Punjabi, Gujarati and Bengali
speakers), Wednesdays 6-10pm
Afro-Carribbean Line: 0800 567 123, Fridays 6-10pm
Minicom service for the hard of hearing: 0800 321 361.

National AIDS Trust
1434 Euston Tower, 286 Euston Road, London NW1 3DN.
Tel: 071-388 1188.

National Children's Bureau
8 Wakley Street, London EC1V 7QE. Tel: 071-278 9441.

National HIV Prevention Information Service
82-86 Seymour Place, London W1H 5DB. Tel: 071-724 7993.

Network of Voluntary Organisations in AIDS/HIV
Health Education Authority. Secretariat: 74 Victoria Crescent,
Glasgow G12 9JQ.

Northern Ireland AIDS Helpline
Room 310, Bryson House, Bedford Street, Belfast BT2 7FE.
Open Mondays, Wednesdays and Fridays 7.30pm till 10pm.
Saturdays 2pm till 5pm. Tel: 0232 326117.

Positive Options
354 Goswell Road, London N1. Tel: 071-278 5039

Positive Partners and Positively Children
Head Office, The Annex, 12-14 Thornton St, London SW9 0BL.
Tel: 071-738 7333.
South London and all of the UK and Ireland.

Positive Partners and Positively Children (continued)
100 Shepherds Walk, London N1 7JN.
Tel: 071-250 1396/0. North London calls.

Positively Women
5 Sebastian St, London EC1V 0HE. Tel: 071-490 5515.

Project for Advice, Counselling and Education
London Lesbian and Gay Centre, 69 Cowcross Street,
London EC1M 6BP. Tel: 071-251 2689.

Red Cross
Contact: Local branch of Red Cross – look in phone book under 'R'
or 'B' (British Red Cross).

Royal National Institute for the Blind
224 Great Portland Street, London W1.
Tel: 071-388 1266.

Save the Children Fund
Mary Datchelor House, 17 Grove Lane, London SE5 8RD.
Tel: 071-703 5400.

Standing Conference on Drug Abuse
1-4 Hatton Place, Hatton Garden, London EC1N 8ND. Tel:
Administration 071-430 2341, Freephone information line Dial 100
for Freephone Drug Problems.

Scottish AIDS Monitor
PO Box 48, Edinburgh EH1 3SA, Scotland. Tel: 031-557 3885.

The Terrence Higgins Trust
52-54 Grays Inn Road, London WC1X 8JU.
Administration: 071-831 0330
Help Line: 071-242 1010 Daily 3-10pm
Vistel for the hard of hearing: 071-405 2463
Daily 7-10pm
Legal Line: 071-405 2381 Wednesdays 7-10pm

Voluntary Council for Handicapped Children
8 Wakley Street, London EC1V 7QE. Tel: 071-278 9441.

Welsh AIDS Campaign
PO Box 348, Cardiff CF1 4XL. Tel: 0222 223443

Index

This index is in word-by-word order. Numbers in **bold** indicate the main source of information; names in **bold** are of bodies cited as pioneering work on HIV/AIDS.